THE MEDICAL TACTICIAN

A century of doctor-patient relationships

Dr Stephen J Connellan

and

'Our Practitioner'

ISBN-10: 1468163469
ISBN-13: 978-1468163469

I dedicate this book to my uncle, Paul
Ignatius Frayne, and 'Our Practitioner'
without whom none of this would have
been possible.

The Medical Tactician

CONTENTS

I am indebted to the British Thoracic Society (Sheila Edwards in particular) for encouragement and support in pursuing publication of this book.

I am grateful to Dr Laurie Slater, Phisick Medical Antiques, for permission to reproduce the pictures of medical equipment.

Instruments courtesy of www.phisick.com

The views expressed and any factual errors presented in this book are entirely my own.

The Medical Tactician

INTRODUCTION

Some 30 years ago my uncle Paul, who was a teacher with a very eclectic literary interest, came across a book in an antiquarian book shop in Liverpool and as I was his only medical professional nephew he gave it to me as a Christmas present. The only identification on the book spine was the title 'Tactics' and written in pencil on the first page "£1". There was no other indication as to the author, publisher or year of writing. The theme was one of doctor-patient relationships and how to achieve success in retaining and increasing the size of one's practice. Advice obtained from the Wellcome Library in London suggests that the original work was a series of articles which the author then bound together with a view to publication. An approximate date of production, based on a number of comments within the text, was during the first decade of the 20th century and therefore out of copyright.

It seems likely that the author was a single-handed medical practitioner who was working in London and whose patients came from a mix of socio-economic backgrounds, which included the wealthy.

I also make the assumption that the author is male. Much of the commentary would support this and in this period of transition between the Victorian and Edwardian eras a female doctor would be much less common. There was still a male dominance in the medical profession and those women, strong and determined enough to practice, were often the subject of prejudice and hostility based on a belief that they would undercut the fees of their male counterparts at a time when there was a glut of practitioners in many of the urban areas.

I have reproduced his type-written work as faithfully as possible, including his use of grammar and underlinings but where there were any obvious spelling errors these have been corrected. There has been some reduction in the number of paragraphs in order to save paper.

The chapters are based on our practitioner's individual articles and I have moved the two chapters on history and examination to the latter sections of the book as these are more tabular and, although still very interesting, stimulate less commentary.

My contribution, whether this is to clarify terms used, enlarge on references to notable historical figures or to add my own experience on doctor-patient relationships, is all in italics.

In the absence of any information as to the original author I refer to him as 'our practitioner'. His approach to the practice of medicine around 1910 provides a fascinating insight in to the challenges, a century ago, facing the equivalent of our current general practitioners. He makes many references to the tactics he uses to gain the confidence of his patients, hence the title of the original compilation of articles. Many of the issues he raises are very relevant to today's medical practice and coping with the sensitivities of the doctor-patient relationship.

His reference to the treatments on offer, equipment used, historical figures and the prevalent diseases of the day, all provide a flavour of what it was like to practice medicine at that time.

I should emphasise at the outset that this is not an academic treatise or critical appraisal of our anonymous practitioner but more a comparison of notes between two doctors who have lived through the ups and downs of medical practice and recognise a certain commonality of experience in the relationship between doctor and patient. References are therefore kept to a minimum and personal anecdotes (sometimes amusing and sometimes scary) help to bring to life the full flavour of what it is/was like to be a practicing doctor in this or the last century.

For a comprehensive and excellent overview of general practice during this period I would recommend:

"The Evolution of British General Practice 1850-1948" by Professor Anne Digby.[1] Her use of archival material, which includes original oral testimony from health care professionals (similar to that provided by 'our practitioner'), provides part of the background for her history of the evolution of general practice over this period.

THE ART OF PRACTICE.

THE INTERVIEW.

By interview is meant the consultation with the patient in the consulting room. Of course it applies also to seeing him at his own house.

Logically this and the article on routine should come after general principles have been discussed. But they contain so many precepts which can be put into practice immediately that they are presented first.

THE IMPRESSIONS TO BE MADE ON THE PATIENT.

1. That you are pleased to see him.

2. That during the interview you are thinking of nothing but the complaint.

3. That you have used every diagnostic means and have overlooked nothing in the inquiry.

4. That you are careful and systematic.

5. That you have had no difficulty in diagnosing the condition.

6. That you take a professional interest.

7. That you take a personal interest.

8. That you are what he calls a "clever" man.

9. That you thoroughly understand him.

10. If the disease is at all distressing that you are sympathetic.

11. That you are sure that you can cure him.

The Medical Tactician

~ CHAPTER 1 ~

THE ART OF PRACTICE

<u>The interview</u>

By interview is meant the consultation with the patient in the consulting room. Of course it applies also to seeing him at his house.

Logically this and the article on routine should come after general principles have been discussed. But they contain so many precepts which can be put into practice immediately that they are presented first.

<u>The impressions to be made on the patient</u>

1) That you are pleased to see him.
2) That during the interview you are thinking of nothing but the complaint.
3) That you have used every diagnostic means and have overlooked nothing in the enquiry.
4) That you are careful and systematic.
5) That you have had no difficulty in diagnosing the condition.
6) That you take a professional interest.
7) That you take a personal interest.
8) That you are what he calls a 'clever ' man.
9) That you thoroughly understand him.
10) If the disease is at all distressing that you are sympathetic.
11) That you are sure that you can cure him.
12) Or at least that you take a cheerful view of the case.
13) That he has found a doctor who inspires cheerfulness and hope.
14) That you are pleased to have had the privilege of seeing him.
15) That he has been treated with all the courtesy and consideration which he (who generally has

a good opinion of himself) thinks is always due
to him.

16)   That he has not taken up more of your time than
you are glad to spare.

The means of producing these impressions

1)   That you are pleased to see him. This is no needless
injunction. You are, in fact, nearly always glad to see a
patient. But do not suppose that he knows it. Patients often
apologise for troubling a doctor. They think he may be
busy, that he wishes to give all his time to other cases, that
he already has so much to do that he is indifferent to a fresh
case, and that perhaps they are taking up time, which the
doctor might like to devote to leisure.

You have yourself sometimes been in a shop where the
tradesman's manner gave the impression that he was
indifferent to seeing you, or was even being ' troubled '. He
was, of course, glad to see you, and your reason told you
this was the case. But you went away with the feeling that
next time he would rather go to some other shop.

The patient must not be left to guess that you are pleased to
see him. He must be shown it. Whatever the social status
of the patient may be, the kindly courteous greeting is due to
him. However solemn you may be by nature, it is quite
within your power to give it if you try. You should always
smile, however artificially. The smile that well bred people
invariably assume when meeting an acquaintance is purely
artificial. But its artificiality jars on no one, and even if the
assumption is obvious, a smile will please the patient and
will not injure your self-respect. Patients often enter the
room in a nervous state. A smile helps as nothing else can
do, to feel more at their ease. It reassures them that they
will be kindly and thoughtfully treated.

Oliver Wendell Holmes has said that a smile may be worth
£1000 a year to a doctor. It costs nothing and will yield a
heavy dividend.

The Medical Tactician

Oliver Wendell Holmes Sr., (August 29, 1809 – October 7, 1894) was a physician by profession but achieved fame as a writer; he was one of the best regarded American poets of the 19th century.

In 1843 he argued that puerperal fever was transmitted from patient to patient by doctors and nurses and his famous essay ' The Contagiousness of Puerperal Fever ' was a forerunner of Pasteur's discovery of the germ theory of disease later in the century.

Another of his quotes was, "Men do not quit playing because they grow old; they grow old because they quit playing."

2)   That during the interview you are thinking of nothing but the complaint. This is the keystone of the arch. It would be difficult to overestimate the necessity for this. Most of the other impressions depend on it. You will never be highly successful if this point is neglected. There must be no acting. Everything but the investigation of the case must be excluded from the mind. Mind-wandering must be checked. If the injunction is followed, the patient will see it quite clearly, and an excellent impression will be made.

3)   That you have used every diagnostic means, and have overlooked nothing. This impression will be made by a good equipment of diagnostic instruments, and by a complete routine examination. These points will be dwelt on elsewhere.

4)   That you are careful and systematic. This will be dealt with under the heading of impressing the patient through the reason.

5)   That you have had no difficulty in diagnosing the condition. The means here are method in examination. This is discussed under the heading of routine. You must school your countenance and manner when an unexpected symptom is mentioned. Do not pause to think over it, as if you were puzzled.

You must talk on as if you were quite familiar with the sign in this particular case. Failure to do this raises doubts in the patient's mind, and a bad effect is produced.

6)   That you take a professional interest. This impression will arise if the interrogation and examination are done in a simple earnest and thoughtful manner, combined with the injunction 2.

7)   That you take a personal interest. This will be given by employing the largest number of therapeutic hints. A very powerful impression can be made in this way. Here a knowledge of treatment other than drugs comes in as most valuable. It rouses the gratitude of the patient, because it shows here that you wish to do more than sell a prescription. That you really have his cure at heart. It convinces the patient also that you know your business. You are compared with the last doctor who failed to advise these little things. He thinks the omission was due to ignorance, or want of interest, and concludes that you are a much superior physician. Such hints are also a strong advertisement. For example, the patient will tell her friends that she is taking hot water before meals, an excellent plan, which she never knew of till she went to doctor X. The name of doctor X. is now advertised for him in a very satisfactory manner.

It is understandable that such a holistic approach to the care of patients a century ago would, to some extent, be driven by the lack of specific curative interventions. However, in spite of the exponential increase in therapeutic intervention, there remains, to this day, a strong drive for alternative and complementary approaches to care.

8)   That you are a 'clever man'. This follows more or less from 3, 5, and other impressions. There are ways of strengthening the effect. When a symptom of indigestion seems probable, you can put the question in an affirmative form. One symptom of indigestion is mentioned. You say, "you have had flatulence, have you not."

The Medical Tactician

The patient thinks you know all about him before asking, which is 'clever'.

<u>Illustrative case</u>

A pale faced young man with a slightly nervous manner calls and complains of an ulcer on the mucous membrane of his cheek, and mentions nothing else. You might examine it carefully, inspect the gums and teeth, advise having any decayed ones removed, recommend a good dentrifice, give a lotion of resorcin, and dismiss him.

Resorcin (or Resorcinol) is a dihydroxy phenol which works as a bactericidal, fungicidal, antipruritic, exfoliative and keratolytic agent. Its properties made it useful in eczematous conditions but our practitioner was presumably recommending it as an antibacterial soothing agent.

You would satisfy him, but you have done nothing to show him that you are 'clever'. His general appearance suggests that he has something else the matter. It might be indigestion. You remark, "you have had indigestion, have you not?" He answers, "yes". Then you interrogate him affirmatively."You have had fullness after meals, I think" etc. His nervous manner suggests neurasthenia. You question him on this. "You have had vague fears, all about nothing?" Probably you have hit the mark, and the answer is again "yes." The patient goes away more than satisfied. He has found a man who knows his work particularly well.

To take another case which is not a suppositious one. A lady fell on the street, and bruised her skin. Next day she sent for a doctor, who was a stranger. No complaint was made except of the local condition. A little nervousness in her manner was suggestive. The doctor suspected she had passed a sleepless night. He found this was the case, and gave a hypnotic, with good result. Had he not enquired beyond the local condition, the patient would not have been dissatisfied, but she would not have been enthusiastic. Her actual remark to a friend was, "I like that man; he knows what he is about."

There may be different pressures on the modern patient but the human psyche has probably not altered much in a century and many modern medics will recognise the scenario of the patient, having completed the consultation, while walking to the door, saying, "Oh by the way Doctor, I'm sure it's nothing but….". Significant pathology may also be accompanied by a confounding psychosomatic element. The patient with well-established asthma, who also suffers with a significant element of hyperventilation or vocal cord dysfunction, broadens the diagnostic dilemma. The diagnosis of pseudo-seizures may be difficult unless an EEG is being performed at the same time. I do recall, however, many years ago, a young man who would always start fitting as the medical team started its ward round. On one occasion, my Consultant drew the curtains around the bed during the fit, leaving us outside. The next thing we heard was a loud slap and a young man's voice shouting, "'ere, wos your game?!" Not to be recommended nowadays of course but an effective diagnostic test!

9)   That you thoroughly understand him. This follows from some of the other impressions, especially that from routine. It is increased by the fact that you have listened carefully to the patient's story <u>without interrupting him</u>. It is increased also by the assured tone of voice in which you say after mention of the symptom, "it is usually so," or "this is nearly always associated." You show by your casual remarks that you are quite familiar with the sign in such cases, and expected to find it present. Should something be mentioned, which at the moment you are unable to account for, you must school your countenance, voice, and manner, to avoid showing you are puzzled.

The pressures of time in modern medicine, whether it be in the GP's surgery, Consultant's outpatient or emergency admissions, have eroded our ability to be good listeners. We are left with a delicate balance of managing throughput without missing the crucial building blocks of a diagnosis. To make matters worse in emergency situations, there is the potential for three doctors of increasing seniority, all with time pressures, asking similar questions, one after the other, of the same patient, without making any diagnostic progress or management plan.

10) If the disease is distressing, that you are sympathetic. If you have not by nature a sympathetic voice, cultivate one as far as you can to do so naturally. If your voice is a loud one, try to subdue it, and speak in a low tone. A loud voice has a jarring effect, and makes it difficult to convey sympathy. If you are not sympathetic by nature, awkward attempts will ring false, and make you ridiculous. But you can at least remark, "I know how disagreeable it is, how painful it is."

Try to put yourself in the patient's place. Imagine his dread or feelings, and your voice will have a truer ring. In any case you can try to comfort him by saying that the symptoms will soon subside, or gently that there is no real cause for alarm, while dwelling on the favourable signs.

In all physical examinations you can be gentle in touch. If you are likely to hurt the patient, even a little, tell him you will be as careful as possible, and then be sure to make your words good.

I can remember, as a medical examiner for the MRCP, wincing on occasions when the candidate set to with a pummelling action on the abdomen without checking to see if the patient was in any way uncomfortable or distressed. Suffice to say the examination was cut short, the candidate given feedback and failure of that section recorded. I was never very keen on including abdominal aortic aneurysms on our list of willing patients!

A natural sympathy is one of the best assets a practitioner can have. The most successful men have possessed it in a high degree. The late Sir Andrew Clarke and the late Sir William Gull were characterised strongly in this quality.

The Medical Tactician

Sir Andrew Clarke (1826-1893) was the son of a doctor from Aberdeen and during his illustrious career he was assistant physician at the city of London Hospital for Diseases of the Chest. He built up a huge reputation both in hospital and private work and became widely acknowledged as a doctor with great powers of observation and scientific approach. He was convinced that many illnesses were the result of poor lifestyle and diet. William Gladstone was one of his most famous patients. In 1888 he became president of the Royal College of physicians until his death due to a stroke.

Sir William Withey Gull, 1st Baronet (1816 – 1890) was elected in 1848 as a Fellow of the Royal College of Physicians. He was also appointed Resident Physician at Guy's and, in a biographical sketch (1896), T.D. Acland records the following passage from the 'Guy's Hospital Reports' which provide a good impression of him.

"His striking presence, his searching scrutiny, his minute and deliberate examination of every case, and the few carefully and slowly uttered words in which he delivered his judgment, sometimes with epigrammatic pungency, often with encouragement, and never without sympathy - all combined to give him an almost unequalled ascendancy over his patients. His manner was his own, and sprang naturally from the habit of his mind. It was just the same in a hospital ward as in a palace, and the poorest of his patients leaned on his oracular statements, sometimes with hope and sometimes with resignation, but always with comfort; while the richest were taught to restrain loquacity, to answer truthfully, and to follow out directions implicitly."

Acland goes on to comment on Gull's healthy cynicism for drug therapy:

"He was never tired of exposing the absurdity of much of the traditional polypharmacy. He would show how much harm may be done by the vigorous treating of half-understood diseases, and he once said that if every drug in

the world were abolished a physician would still be a useful member of society. To appreciate his position, we must remember something of the unquestioning faith in bleeding and blistering, purging and physicking, which was still held when Gull was a student."

Gull would be dismayed to see the number of elderly patients now admitted to hospital as a direct result of polypharmacy!

In the words of Sir Frederick Treves, "The physician must be kind. He must needs be a man of wide sympathy, and be able to put himself in the patient's place."

Sir Frederick Treves, 1st Baronet (1853-1923) was a surgeon, specialising in abdominal surgery, at the Royal London Hospital. As Sergeant Surgeon to King Edward VII he saved the King's life by operating on his perforated appendix. Around 1886 Treves brought Joseph Carey Merrick, 'the Elephant Man', to the London Hospital where Merrick lived until he died in 1890. Treves founded the Red Cross Society and was a life-long friend of Thomas Hardy. Ironically, he died as a result of a perforated appendix at the age of 70 years.

If for no other reason but your own success, try to cultivate the quality. There have been men lacking in most of the necessary characteristics, but who have had a natural sympathy, and they have been moderately successful.

11)   That you are sure that you can cure him. If the case is one in which you are reasonably sure that the recovery will be made, don't dismiss the patient till you have said so confidently. Remark in a cheerful voice, not that you think or hope he will soon be well, but say with a simple assurance, "you will soon get all right."

12)   Or at least that you take a cheerful view of the case. If you are doubtful about the course the case may take, dwell on the good points.

Mention for example, that the heart and lungs are sound, that the open air life led is an advantage etc. Ignore the unfavourable conditions.

13)   That he has found a doctor who inspires cheerfulness and hope. This follows from 9, 11 and 12. The impression can be reinforced by manner. This will be referred to under another heading.

14)   That you are pleased to have had the privilege of seeing him. This follows from the courtesy of reception, and dismissal, from the other impressions, and from showing no signs of a hurry.

15)   That he has been treated with all the courtesy which is due to him. This follows from the above impressions and avoiding certain mistakes which are referred to elsewhere.

16)   That he has taken up no more of your time than you are glad to spare. This follows as in 14, and from the fact that you have never interrupted his story. At the dismissal the smile is once more imperative.

Additional remarks on the interview

Never under any circumstances talk about extraneous subjects till the prescription has been given. If the patient introduces a relevant matter, do not interrupt immediately. If she continues, tactfully divert the conversation back to the illness. If, after the prescription stage, she wishes to chat, be a good listener only. If the patient is a social equal, and you are a little friendly, the rule may be relaxed somewhat. But do no more than is necessary to avoid appearing unsociable. It is wise never to talk about yourself, however trivial or innocent the remark may be. It is important to show no special interest in anything. The reason for this is discussed elsewhere. Avoid making any enquiry after prescribing. Should you do so you have failed in systematic method. The patient sees this and thinks he has been prescribed for without a full examination.

The Medical Tactician

A garrulous patient may interrupt the routine. Avoid showing any annoyance. Try tactfully to bring the conversation back to the desired channel. If she talks about the weather, seem to think of it in relation to her illness, and reply in this sense. Then get on with the examination. You may be able to check the flow of language by asking her to put out her tongue, by counting her pulse with moving lips, or similar methods. After the prescription stage, listen, if you can spare the time, but without any remark that might lead to further talk. If you are really pressed for time, or if other patients are waiting, talk yourself for a few seconds, and then stand up, as if you consider the interview at an end.

Don't show a patient a book, or quote from one. They like to think you're treating them from your own knowledge and experience alone. You might convey the idea that you have not the necessary knowledge to deal with the case.

The roles are now often reversed since the empowerment of patients with Internet search engines. Some will research all aspects of their condition, occasionally on less reliable sites, and wait to see if the doctor has knowledge of the condition which is as up-to-date as theirs. Comprehensive overviews will naturally worry patients as they are likely to assume that all aspects of the condition will apply to them.

There are two exceptions, one where the patient thinks he has been wrongly treated, and the other is where an unfavourable result is likely to occur. For example, if stiffness after Colles fracture happens, you will escape blame if you have pointed out this possibility in black and white. But some suspicion might remain if you had merely given warning. It might be thought that you had only done so to cover your want of skill.

During the evolutionary process of our relationship with patients we have eschewed the paternalistic approach and Governance has ensured that consent to interventions is fully informed. Gone is the hand on the shoulder accompanied by the words, "You let me worry about that!"

The Medical Tactician

We have decided that it is essential that the worry is shared between the patient and the responsible health professional. This accepted advance in honest doctor-patient relationships is inevitably more difficult to manage and more stressful for both parties.

If you give a new drug don't tell the patient so. Don't say it is the latest product from Germany. Patients don't wish to be treated with new drugs. They wish to think they are getting the results of your own experience. The same caution applies to advice and not connected with drugs. For similar reasons don't give a sample bottle of medicine.

You must school your countenance, and not even seem to smile when told of aneroids in the throat, or paradise of the legs.

The patient's expertise in malapropisms will never wane and many of us will have had to 'school our countenance' following such statements delivered with considerable gravitas. I recall an elderly lady (around the time of the Falkland's war) bemoaning the fact that her new GP wouldn't prescribe those excellent 'Exocet' suppositories for her Rheumatoid arthritis and couldn't help but muse on the spectre of this heat-seeking device targeting her rectum. I once overheard a couple asking a man, standing outside a hospital department, if this was the infertility clinic. The sign above the door said 'Sterile Supplies'! Other reported classics include:

Family member to paramedic... "We've been doing cardio-preliminary resurrection for about 10 minutes now."

"I can't take a water pill, it messes up my electric lights."

"A child with eczema had crustaceans in his ears."

A medical student was asked where you find men with XYY chromosomes, her response was: "In penile institutions."

It is not worthwhile explaining when a patient tells you that a doctor took out her mother's eye for examination, and put it back again. Never do such a thing as to deceive the patient about the amount of pain you are about to inflict. Don't tell him you will not hurt him, and then plunge a knife in his abscess. You would incur both resentment and loss of confidence.

Commonly heard euphemistic phrases that trip off the doctor's tongue may be heard in all departments and include, "Just a little prick," "Just a little scratch," "This shouldn't hurt too much." Best avoided when attempting arterial blood gases on a patient with wobbly and hardened radial arteries. Local anaesthetic isn't very expensive. One of the main reasons put forward by asthmatics for not wanting to be readmitted with acute asthma was the fear of having to have arterial blood gases.

Do not try to talk a patient out of her sufferings. You are likely to be thought either indifferent or unsympathetic.

When reassuring an alarmed patient, do not do so in an ordinary tone of voice. You must adopt a special, earnest, and emphatic manner, and say the symptoms have no unfavourable significance. But while being earnest and emphatic, do not overdo it; else you will have the appearance of insincerity or affectation.

Reassure the patient as to the duration of the illness, and your ability to relieve the pain. Dwell on the favourable features of the case, such as, that he is not old, and has a good constitution, etc.

Even if the patient is not alarmed, do not forget to say you can relieve the symptoms.

This may be taken for granted if not expressed. But the effect is much greater if a confident statement is made.

When asking delicate questions, do so in as simple and natural a manner as you can, as if professional life had made you hardened to the matter. Use as refined language as circumstances permit, but avoid circumlocution.

In requesting exposure of the lower part of the person, remember that modesty is not always the cause of reluctance. This may be due to a desire not to expose soiled linen. If the patient comes with psoriasis of the arms, and you ask to look at the knees, and hesitation is shown, say at once, "never mind, it is hardly necessary."

A more modern reluctance to undress may be a regretted tattoo such as that revealed to me after reassurance that breast examination was essential in her case. Under the left nipple was tattooed, 'mild' and under the right 'bitter.'

Cultural differences in predominantly female modesty are not considered by our practitioner but this may be because his practice was almost exclusively white caucasian.

In suggesting delicate examinations, it is well to hint first that this is necessary. The reluctance diminishes with time, and it will be submitted to more willingly at a future period. It is better not to leave it to be understood that a third person must be present. Mention it yourself, then do your best to fulfil your promise not to cause pain. Give all directions together at the prescription stage. Do not give them by instalments. You cannot be too clear about this matter. Except in the simplest cases, write them down. This is seldom done even by very successful men, but it is well worth the time and trouble. It is an advertisement for you which will be commented on. You will get a reputation for carefulness. Medical men little know how minutely they are discussed, that every trifling action is noticed and gossiped about. They occasionally hear of it when there is an imputation against skill, or in the case of exaggerated praise. Beyond such they usually hear nothing. Rely on it that if you write down instructions, the patient's friends will hear of it.

In spite of the passage of 100 years this important advice is still not widely adhered to. Many an audit of inpatient care of acute asthma will reveal a lack of any written management plan on discharge. The use of drawings to explain medical concepts is much appreciated by patients and better retained than verbal description.

Written advice is particularly important in the case of informed consent. The Defence unions' back catalogues are littered with cases in which the patient hadn't been advised of the potential risks of a procedure.

There is another reason. Patients forget much more easily than you think, and remembering is more difficult than you would imagine. For example, when telling a patient how to make a linseed-meal poultice, the patient understands at the time and then goes home and forgets whether the water is to be added to the meal, or the meal to the water.

Mrs Beeton's Household Management describes the production of linseed-meal poultice as follows:

' Scald your basin, by pouring a little hot water into it, then put a small quantity of finely ground linseed meal into the basin, pour a little hot water on it and stir it around briskly until you have well incorporated them, add a little more meal and a little more water, then stir it again. Do not let any lumps remain in the basin but stir the poultice well and do not be sparing of your trouble. What you do next, is to take as much of it out of the basin as you may require, lay it on a piece of soft linen, and let it be about a quarter of an inch thick .'

Mustard was often added to this mixture and the resultant poultice used to bring boils to a head, relieve swollen joints and ease chest complaints by spreading over the area that was presumed to be inflamed.

The late Sir Andrew Clark, who was a very busy man, never omitted to write his directions. He was an excellent master of tactics. He wrote in red ink. This is a good plan. It helps the patient to identify the paper if put among others. A very little thing like this will be noted and commented on.

Many surgical colleagues continue the practice of using red ink to indicate operation notes but the downside may be poor reproduction when notes are copied for medico-legal reasons.

This recommendation to write directions comes from patients who have been disgusted at forgetting what they were told to do. Elsewhere it is inculcated that patients are unreasonable, and do not make allowances. If a direction is forgotten, there will be a feeling of irritation against you.

Explanation of advice

When recommending something, do not give the scientific reason why. The association of two ideas, the thing recommended, and the good it will do, becomes fixed by a wave of conviction, resulting from the confident manner in which you gave it. Any explanation only weakens the effect. For example, when saying that baked potatoes agree better than boiled ones, don't explain that the heat of the oven breaks open the starch granules, and makes these more digestible.

Even in the case of a well-educated man, it is better to avoid explaining therapeutics. The wisdom implied from the admonition is magnified, and is only diminished by disclosing the rationale, just as a conjurors trick seems less wonderful when we know how it is done.

When in giving a diagnosis - a patient says she has never had such a thing before, and that her family have never had such a thing; reply, that every event must have a first time, that she is only human, and that she is liable to human infirmities.

No incredulity should be shown at untrue statements. There is one exception. When a patient mentions symptoms which you are sure she does not feel, show by ignoring them that she is not believed. But do nothing more than ignore them.

Medical practitioners will recognise the outpatient scenario in which the patient sits next to you at an angle to the desk. Just within view is the accompanying carer, relative/friend sitting in the corner of the room but making sure that he or she can gesticulate furiously to you when they think that the patient is providing wrong/exaggerated information or underplaying symptoms. This is always tricky because there is no guarantee that the gesticulator isn't actually dementing themselves. A good GP referral letter is worth its weight in gold in such circumstances.

Never laugh at a patient. In one case only may it be done. If she shows a superstitious disinclination to admit that she is better, laugh (genially) and let her see she is not believed.

Never interrupt a patient. You must listen to nonsense just as carefully as if what he was saying were important.

In the article on routine it is enjoined that a great number of questions should be asked at the first interview, whether these are necessary or not, (in ordinary cases). Make a practice of not omitting to ask three questions, as to sleep, appetite, state of the bowels, and of not omitting to feel the pulse and to look at the tongue.

These five points may not be necessary, but remember that the patient does not know this, and they think they are. Therefore never forget them. The impression made the first time a patient sees you is much stronger and much more lasting than at any other subsequent occasion. The reason why is obscure. The fact remains that such is the case. If for good, even mistakes in the future may be overlooked, if for bad, it is difficult to make up for lost ground. If a good first impression is combined with a favourable progress of the case, you are likely to get lifelong friends, who will become your enthusiastic advertisers. Redouble, if possible, your efforts with each fresh patient you see. It must not be implied however that carelessness in subsequent interviews will have no effect.

Attention

We have said above that giving the whole attention to the case is the keystone of the arch. It is easy to give this advice. To carry it out is another matter. The flood of thoughts that keep welling up have to be combated. With some people this is moderately easy. With the majority it is very difficult.

The question is of such importance that it is worthwhile considering what can be done to cure mind-wandering.

Concentration, if present, is clear to the patient. It inspires confidence in gratitude. If not present, the absence is also clear to the patient. It is not possible to simulate it.

The practitioner who has concentration naturally bestowed starts with a great advantage. He is pretty certain to be moderately successful, even if lacking in other desirable qualities. The truth of this is a matter of observation.

First let us consider what militates against concentration, leaving aside the question of habitual mind-wandering.

There are three chief factors. 1. Worry. 2. Faulty respiration. 3. Muscular strain.

1) A worried man cannot concentrate. This need not be further discussed. There is no recipe to be given for guarding against worry.

2) Faulty respiration. This can be guarded against. A huddled up posture can be avoided, and long breaths will help.

3)   Muscular strain can be reduced to a minimum. The easiest posture that circumstances allow can be chosen. There is no need to stand up, when a chair can be used.

I would add to this, profound exhaustion. The working hours of doctors has been greatly improved in recent years (some would say it has gone too far with the consequence that practical experience and education are suffering). During my 6 months as a Medical House Officer we were expected to work a 120 hour week on a 1:2 rota. If your colleague went off sick you were back on call. I can remember a sort of euphoric trance-like state towards the end of a Monday evening having been continually on-call since the preceding Friday morning. Thankfully that is all part of history but modern doctors will still be working for around 50 hours per week and more when the demands of preparing teaching sessions, dealing with enormous amounts of administration (including the additional bureaucracy that comes with medical management and governance) are taken in to consideration. So patients shouldn't be surprised when the doctor taking their history desperately tries to stifle a yawn but just ends up appearing to be in training for a national gurning competition.

The above advice, necessary as it is, only does a little. What else can be done?

Professor James says: "Try to attend steadfastly to a dot on a paper, or on the wall. Either your vision becomes blurred, or your eye wanders away to something else. But if you ask yourself questions about the dot, how big it is, how far, of what shape, what shade or colour, etc., you can keep your mind on it for a comparatively long time."

What can be done with a simple thing, can be done with something less simple, such as the interrogation and examination of patients. Constant self questioning can be carried out. For example, you can say to yourself, "this patient's organs are all sound, why is he ill at all?"

The Medical Tactician

One constant question should be asked, 'Am I systematic? Am I finding out all there is to learn about this patient?' Interest should be excited. Speculate about the condition. For example, say to yourself, 'what is the reason this patient is always breaking down in health? '

A highly successful man once said: "I look on every case as I would on a game of chess." Try to regard every case as a problem, about which everything has to be found out. Get out of the habit of looking at patients with typical symptoms as a type. Every patient is atypical in some respect.

I once overheard a junior doctor in the on-call room say, "The next patient has COPD. I might as well start writing the history down now."

Never be satisfied with half success in concentration. After each patient has left the room, ask yourself the question: 'did I exclude everything extraneous from the mind during the examination?' If the answer is 'no', be dissatisfied till the answer is always 'yes'.

It is certain that concentration can be greatly strengthened by practice. Here maybe mention the importance of cultivating the power of observation. How badly this quality is usually developed, is shown by the clock test referred to in the prospectus. The first necessity is to keep your eyes open. The majority of people do not. The power of observation can be enormously increased by practice. Houdini trained himself by glancing at shop windows, till at last he could note and remember everything in the window by a single glance.

You can practise the habit on the street. Give one rapid look at someone you pass. Try to see what you have noted as to his dress, gait, features, etc. Practice with shop windows, your own sideboard, mantelpiece, pictures, etc.

The story is told of Agassiz. He gave a student a fish to describe. The student wrote a report in 10 minutes. Agassiz refused to take it. He kept the student at the fish for three days, before he was even moderately satisfied.

Jean Louis Rodolphe Agassiz (1807-1873) was a Swiss-American zoologist, glaciologist, and geologist and one of the first world-class American scientists. He made significant discoveries regarding glaciers and found that they moved after driving a line of stakes across one and observing it bend.

In 1842-1846 he issued his Nomenclator Zoologicus, a comprehensive classified list of all genera and groups employed in zoological reference.

~ CHAPTER 2 ~

ROUTINE AND EXAMINATION OF PATIENTS

This is part of the whole subject, influencing patients through the Reason. It is here given out of its order.

A certain practitioner preferred as a locum a newly qualified man, to one more experienced. His reason was that the former, fresh from the wards of a hospital, had not got out of the habit of routine examination, and this routine gave great satisfaction to the patients.

It is to be feared that many practitioners fall into the habit of attending to the essential, and leaving the apparently unessential.

This is injudicious. Frequently unsuspected things can be discovered. Patients often omit important symptoms. Women are often afraid to volunteer certain statements, and hope they will be asked on them. If not, they go away dissatisfied.

I suspect that this related more to the fact that medical practitioners were predominantly men. I wonder if women opened up more on their problems when more women doctors started practicing.

The effect of a full interrogation and examination is strong. It shows that the case is being fully investigated, and confidence is given. It conveys the impression that a professional and personal interest are being taken.

If the practitioner can go through the routine systematically, and without hesitation, the patient thinks he knows his business well. Though she is silent to you on the impression made, depend on it, the carefulness will be mentioned to many others, with the additional remark, that you are 'clever', and in some cases a comparison with the care taken by another doctor will be discussed in a wide circle.

The Medical Tactician

I recall the stethoscope choreography of a certain highly respected Senior Physician during my medical student days. The diaphragm end would be waved ceremoniously in front of the patient's face then very lightly touched, in rapid succession, to various parts of the body with a rather camp upward flip after contact. Either he had superhuman acoustic acumen or he was relying on the consensus view of his entourage. In any event, I'm sure that the patient was impressed at his thoroughness. Always useful to have a team in support. Not a luxury provided to our intrepid practitioner.

The subtleties of clinical examination have, through the intervening years, been undermined by our more sophisticated investigative armament. Gone are the days when there might be discussion as to whether there was a 4th heart sound present or a little flurry of excitement on hearing whispering pectoriloquy (never mind spelling it). It's a brave clinician who will claim classical aegophony on auscultation without having a quick sneak at the chest x-ray!

Not all men realise the legitimate advertisement they can get by thorough routine. The following was the reputation of a practitioner in a London suburb.

"He is very good as a rule, but careless with children". This man was evidently not systematic in examination, and the omission must have cost him a considerable diminution of practice.

A proper routine comprises negative, as well as positive investigation. It is often as important to find out that there is no oedema of the legs as to ascertain that there is.

The inquiry should be comprehensive. If conducted along the line of the patient's complaints only, but little light is thrown, and important points may be overlooked. A thorough examination is hardly possible unless system and routine are followed.

After the preliminary entries in the case-book of name, age, occupation, and address, the inquiry is divided into interrogation and physical examination. Interrogation comes first.

It is interesting to note the use of the word interrogation which nowadays has more of a connotation of officialdom and potential serious consequences. The word is derived from the Latin interrogare, to question, so seems appropriate. When did doctors start 'taking a history'? Many centuries before but it was certainly in use in 1899 as demonstrated by the book, 'The Elements of Clinical Diagnosis' by Georg Klemperer [2] in which he states, "A diagnosis is reached by the examination of the patient. This consists in the obtaining of the history (anamnesis) and in the objective examination (status praesens)."

By the way, if you would prefer to use these older descriptors then you would surely be tempted by 'heteroanamnesis' which is obtaining history from someone else who knows the patient!

INTERROGATION

The first question should be 'what do you complain of?' not, 'what is the matter?' The patient often takes this to mean 'what is the diagnosis?', and may reply 'that is what I came to find out,' and may afterwards boast of his good retort.

Let him tell his story in his own way. <u>NEVER INTERRUPT.</u> Then ask the duration, and whether the onset was gradual or sudden, what was noticed first, what the order was in the appearance of the symptoms, and which are causing most trouble. Has he been under other treatment, and if so, what was done.

Our Practitioner is of course rightly pointing out the need to be a good listener in all our consultations. There is, however, the occasional heart-sink situation that arises when a patient unfolds a fully typed manuscript outlining, in fine detail, the many and varied symptoms, chronology, their own personal view as to the causation and a comprehensive background literature search from the internet.

One approach in such circumstances is to pre-empt with the question, "What would you say is the thing that most concerns you at present?" You may get an interesting response such as, "I'm going through a very stressful divorce," which may add useful extra insight in to the patient's overall presentation.

Finally, always thank the patient very much for taking the time and effort to produce such a comprehensive document, ask if you can file it in their notes, emphasising that you will use it as a supplement to this consultation and then move on to direct history taking. Perusal of the document while dictating your letter will probably be more beneficial to the patient in the long run.

Take next the family history, the condition of immediate relatives, if living, or cause of death, if not. The inquiry should include the patient's children, if any.

Then comes the personal history. Ask exact nature of occupation, home surroundings, exercise taken, food, alcohol and tobacco, quality and amount.

Some doctors seem to have a bit of a blind spot when it comes to occupational history. They don't fully appreciate the proportion of a patient's life that may be in potentially hazardous environments with all the implications of dust, fumes, chemicals, allergens, environmental extremes and stress. To record in the notes 'Retired' with no further comment is poor practice.

Our practitioner makes no reference to any known allergies and I suspect that this was a field of medicine that was somewhat 'embryonic' at the time. In fact the scientific interest in allergy really took off around 1910. The potential for drug allergies was much less, for obvious reasons. Bela Schick described allergy in terms of serum sickness in 1905 and Clemens von Pirque [3], coined the term 'allergy' in 1906 to describe all forms of 'altered reactivity' which we now think of as allergic diseases such as asthma, hay fever and urticaria.

At a time when physicians commonly considered asthma to be a disease of the central nervous system, Samuel Meltzer (1851-1920) [4] introduced the idea that asthma was the result of an immunological response. He applied the new concept of hypersensitivity, to explain asthma and his laboratory experiments, detailing the physiological reaction of anaphylaxis in guinea pigs, supported his claims. He subsequently publicised his views in a landmark address to the Association of American Physicians in 1910.

An Italian Professor, Bernardino Ramazzini [5] described occupational health hazards in 52 working environments in 1713. His description of the sufferings of grain workers was as follows: "Almost all who make a living by sifting or measuring grain are short of breath and cachectic and rarely reach old age; in fact, they are very liable to lapse into orthopnoea and finally dropsy." He was describing the natural history of hypersensitivity pneumonitis but it wasn't until 1932 that J Munro Campbell [5] linked this presentation to agricultural workers and mouldy hay.

There is no mention of pets either and it probably wasn't appreciated that domestic pets could be a source of disease whether it be due to allergic reactions or infections.

The previous health should then be gone into. Inquire what former illnesses there have been, and in a man often a direct question may be made as to specific disease. In a woman, question on the symptoms only, loss of hair, sore throat etc.

Interesting sensitivities once again demonstrated in his dealings with women patients. I suspect that asking one of his female patients if they have ever suffered with Syphilis (referred to as specific disease by our practitioner) would not have gone down very well and reduced his income significantly. I'm not convinced that many doctors nowadays routinely ask their new patients, male or female, whether they have suffered any form of sexually transmitted disease (STD) or even, in the relevant cases, what their sexual preferences are.

I trained at St Mary's Hospital, London and as medical students we had the opportunity to see plenty of STDs in the 'Special Clinic' and some quite dramatic sequelae of earlier Syphilis. This unit was situated in the basement but is now at street level and deals with Sexual Health. I recall an Italian, whose English was not perfect, who presented to one of the clinics we attended. He passed a piece of paper to our Consultant who then passed it round to us. On it was written, 'I think I am having the venerable disease'. He was correct in his assumption although I'm not convinced that his recent sexual history was worthy of reverence.

In the following interrogation of each functional system, the order is immaterial, but the practitioner should always keep to the same.

If the complaint is to a particular system, the inquiry should be on this first, and the special scheme should be used. Then the general scheme should be gone into, and if any fresh symptom is discovered, the special interrogation should be employed once more.

There follows a comprehensive section on history taking and the medical examination which I have decided to move to the final chapters of the book,(7 & 8), not because I feel that the reader will be less interested but because these sections are in more tabular form with less in the way of commentary. Clinicians will be interested for their own specialties, to see how much detail is gone in to, the different emphasis in some cases and the omissions compared with modern day history taking.

The section on clinical examination of both adults and children, although biased to the prevalent diseases of the day, would act as a very satisfactory tutorial for any training physicians, even though it is 100 years old!

Any readers with no medical training may prefer to skip the last 2 chapters and move on to the epilogue but may equally be interested in the approach to history taking and examination of patients.

~ CHAPTER 3 ~

GENERAL REMARKS

Often in business the one principle to keep in mind is to give the customer what he wants and not what is believed he ought to have. The great catering industry built up by Sir Joseph Lyons, who caters for over half a million people daily and who has nearly 16,000 employees, has been made a success by holding to this one end.

Sir Joseph Lyons (1848-1917), British caterer, began by catering at public exhibitions. He next opened tea-shops in London, the first in 1894; 20 years later these numbered over 200 and provided cheap food for the large class of clerical workers and junior members of professions. He died in London in 1917. Our Practitioner's comments above, which suggest Sir Joseph is still living, would seem to support the assumption that he was writing this in the first or early second decade of the 1900s.

Theatre managers have learnt this lesson, sometimes by sad experience. While in business this principle is often the sole factor, in medical practice it is always the sole factor. The apparent exceptions are found not to be exceptions.

It would appear that our Practitioner was espousing patient choice well before all our political parties have made this part of their manifestos in recent times.[7] However, it is somewhat more complicated in the modern scenario, with real choice being thwarted to some degree by expectation outstripping resource and geographical considerations. Attempts at informed choice also remain challenging as a result of suboptimal data quality.

There might seem no object in pointing this out, because it leaves the question "What is it patients want?" At first sight it appears similar to saying to a chess learner, "Make the right moves and you will win," or to a beginner in music, "Strike the right notes in the right time."

It is not so useless as it seems. It keeps the inquiry in the right channel. If the question "What does the patient want?" is fully answered, all the conditions for success in practice are fully known.

Patients themselves instinctively classify two qualities that they desire. They call these 'Clever' and 'Nice. To the word "Nice" they attach a much wider meaning than that of ordinary use.

The impression of ability ('cleverness') is dealt with under the heading of 'Impressing patients through the reason,' and the means of producing the desired effect is shown.

Real ability does little to give the impression if the means recommended are not followed. Many a man who does not deserve it is called clever. Many a man who does deserve it is not. The explanation lies partly in the inherent difficulty which patients have in judging of knowledge and skill.

The real ability of a chess player or a billiard player is easy to see. That of a medical man is not. A further fallacy comes in. The 'nice' man who has moderate knowledge of impressing patients through the reason has his 'cleverness' magnified through the bias created by his 'niceness.'

How this latter impression can be conveyed is dealt with under the headings of –

'Impressing Patients through the Aesthetic Faculties'

'Impressing Patients through the Emotions and Tact.'

Before examining the psychology of patients, a little self-inspection is desirable.

A very successful man requires no persuading that it is necessary to study very closely the patient's point of view, that small things are of much importance, and that the factors are numerous.

His sympathetic knowledge of human nature has told him this. The unsuccessful man is also willing to admit that he has much to learn. He knows it by sad experience. The moderately successful man is more difficult to convince. He generally has some of the necessary qualities naturally bestowed, but his insight in to human nature has its limits. He thinks there is no region beyond his own vision. What success he has makes him more or less satisfied, and he never reflects that there are a hundred ways in which he could increase his practice. But the sight of others doing much better ought to make him see that there is a cause of some kind and that such a cause is worth investigating. He usually ascribes the greater success of others to luck or 'personality.' It can be shown, however, by facts that 'personality' is harmful, except when it embodies certain desirable qualities.

The following is a concrete example of a fairly successful practitioner. He was an excellent therapeutist and had a good knowledge of medical science. If he had had nothing more than this he would have been a complete failure, but he was gifted with cheerfulness and confidence. He was moderately successful. He would have been highly so if he had not violated almost every rule enjoined in this course. He had no insight into human nature and never looked at things from the patient's point of view.

The moderately successful men are instructive, because they show that many qualities are necessary for complete success. A man with a brusque manner or one with a chilling manner may make a bare living by certain other good qualities, but the repelling influence has an effect and limits success.

Our Practitioner, in common with many of his colleagues, was in private medicine. Hence the common thread which strives to retain patients and make a good living. One wonders if our contemporary colleagues who do both NHS and private work adopt a different persona when working in the private sector. It is said that the more successful private practitioners earned their reputation first and foremost by the feedback from patients and GPs during their initial practice in the NHS. It is potentially easier to be 'patient friendly' in private consulting rooms because there is less time pressure and the surroundings may be more comfortable. Doctors are human beings with all the associated frailties and modern medicine puts them under enormous pressure at times, which may bring out the darker side of their character. This may be more difficult to suppress in an overbooked clinic, with a teaching commitment, inexperienced junior support requiring help throughout, and another important commitment looming ahead with no sign of the clinic finishing on time. There are, however, far fewer 'characters' in hospital medicine than in earlier years; Governance and 360 degree appraisal, where practiced, have controlled this aspect to some extent. One of my colleagues in an earlier existence would sneak a quick cigarette during clinic and if you caught him at the wrong moment you would notice a little plume of smoke emanating from the top drawer where the ash tray was hidden! I suspect any attempt to pursue this now would result in a thorough dowsing with a fire extinguisher and a reminder to attend the next Fire lecture.

There is also the risk of familiarity breeding contempt and I remember an Obs and Gynae Consultant who was coming to the end of his career having lost his bed side manner somewhere along the way. Having inserted a speculum he bent down to inspect and after a brief pause exclaimed, "Oh my God!" stood up slowly and beckoned to the students to follow him to a discrete distance where he informed them that his car had slipped its brake that morning and he had ricked his back 'something awful' while trying to stop it. One of the students nipped back quickly to release the lady from the ceiling and reassure her that all was well.

Some people believe that some of our stronger characteristics, whether benign or malignant, become more accentuated as we get older and perhaps this is something we need to be aware of in our colleagues as they approach retirement.

The Medical Tactician

Our Practitioner will of course have his own stresses relating to maintaining his patient list and life style whereas our contemporary colleagues, whether in primary or secondary care, enjoy a good salary and pension (at least for the time being).

It is almost self-evident that the question must be approached from the patient's point of view. What is necessary to grasp and keep in mind is that this point of view is not the same as that of the doctor. For example, a practitioner knows that a bottle with an untidy wrapper will do as much good as one neatly done up. But he must recognise that a patient is influenced by such small matters and will in some cases form a sweeping judgment upon them. She may think that the doctor who is careless in this is careless generally.

THE PATIENT'S IDEAL

Two main divisions show themselves at once. The sick person wants to be cured. The first requirement is skill. To possess knowledge is not enough. There is an art in showing that it is possessed. When a patient buys coal she cares for nothing but quality and price. When she buys medical skill she wants the presence of certain attracting qualities and the absence of certain repelling ones, i.e. positive and negative attributes.

The positive are -

1. The ability to give confidence in the power to cure. Implicated in this are decision, self-reliance, courage, firmness, certainty. Cheerfulness comes under this heading also. The effect is a compound one. It implies success in achieving what is attempted. The man who wins at a game or succeeds in business is generally more cheerful than the man who fails. Therefore this quality suggests success and gives confidence. Secondly it is contagious. A pleasant state of mind is conveyed.

Distinctiveness in speaking and giving orders. The impression is given that the doctor knows what he is about.

2. The power to allay fears
3. The ability to convey sympathy (in certain cases). The effect here is compound. Often a patient wants sympathy and is dissatisfied if she does not get it. Therefore it gives the idea that the doctor who is sympathetic will do his best. Hence the feeling of confidence.
4. Honesty, and with it is associated candour.
5. Naturalness. Simplicity.
6. Gentleness in touch, gentleness in everything.
7. Brevity. By this is meant that while the fullest examination is made with no signs of hurry, it should be so systematic that no time is wasted. The patient should see that the doctor has system and routine and that she will not be bored by an interview unnecessarily long.
8. Dignity. Self-respect.
9. Trustworthiness. This is a compound of honesty and ability
10. Personal equation. This is dwelt on under the aesthetic faculties and emotions.

The negative are −

1. Conceit. Vanity
2. Depression. Ill temper
3. Pompousness. Too much solemnity
4. Verbosity
5. Artificiality. Affectation
6. Hurry. Impatience

To give the above list and leave it without exposition would be of little use.

Confidence and the means of producing it are discussed under the 'Interview,' 'The Sick Room,' 'Routine,' etc.

The qualities that are harmful, those of the second list, are chiefly negative of the first. The qualities that appeal most or repel most are not the same to all people. For example, brusqueness is much more resented by some than by others. Further, the psychology of women is different from that of men. Women are much more impressionable through the emotional and aesthetic faculties. They are much more easily attracted and are easier to convince, though they see through insincerity more readily. They are far more observant and pay greater attention, and attach more importance to detail. From instinct and long practice they take in every small matter without appearing to do so. They observe everything in your house, everything in your dress, deportment, manner, at a glance. They often judge more by the tone of voice than by the words spoken. They watch your face as very few practitioners realise, but without appearing to do so. They are much more influenced by price. They have a much finer artistic sense and with them the personal equation comes in very strongly.

Weir Mitchell remarks: - "A man may be a competent, clear headed, scrupulously careful doctor, and fail because he is plain or ill-dressed."

Our Practitioner was presumably influenced by the writings of Silas Weir Mitchell who was an eminent American Physician and writer (1829 -1914) [8] who also commented on the doctor patient relationship and the psyche of women. It is worth considering an abstract from one of his published essays in 'Doctor and Patient' (published by J B Lippincott Company in 1888), to get the full flavour of his thoughts on women.

"I have often been asked by ill women if my contact with the nervous weaknesses, the petty moral deformities of feminine nature, had not ,lessened my esteem for woman. I say, surely, no! So much of these is due to educational errors, so much to false relationships with husbands, so much is born out of that which healthfully dealt with, or fortunately surrounded, goes to make all that is sincerely charming in

the best of women. The largest knowledge finds the largest excuses, and therefore no group of men so truly interprets, comprehends, and sympathises with woman as do physicians, who know how near to disorder and how close to misfortune she is brought by the very peculiarities of her nature, which evolve in health the flower and fruitage of her perfect life. With all her weaknesses, her unstable emotionality, her tendency to morally warp when long nervously ill, she is then far easier to deal with, far more amenable to reason, far more sure to be comfortable as a patient than the man who is relatively in a like position"
...... He goes on to say .. "The woman's desire to be on a level of competition with man and to assume his duties is, I am sure, making mischief, for it is my belief that no length of generations of change in her education and modes of activity will ever alter her characteristics. She is physiologically other than man."

It was also Weir Mitchell who promoted the 'Rest Cure' for mental disorders, (particularly hysteria), which was essentially strict bed rest, exclusion from family contact and a fatty diet. It was almost always prescribed to women, many of whom were suffering from depression. It was not effective and caused many to go insane or die! Need there be any further commentary on the distorted mental machinations of this man.

Charlotte Perkins Gilman [9] a feminist writer, performer and activist, was one of Mitchell's patients. She wrote a story about a woman (based on her own experience) who suffers from mental illness after three months of being closeted in a room by her husband for the sake of her health. She was forbidden to touch a pen, pencil or brush ever again, and only allowed two hours of stimulation a day. She is nearly driven mad by the room's revolting yellow wallpaper. She wrote this story to change people's minds about the role of women in society, and emphasised that women's lack of autonomy was detrimental to their mental, emotional, and even physical wellbeing.

Everything in the 'Rest Cure' that Mitchell prescribed ruled out any mental stimulation and, in the story, she was essentially kept by her husband in solitary confinement. Her story, 'The Yellow Wallpaper', published in the January 1892 issue of The New England Magazine, was essentially a response to Mitchell and she sent him a copy. It is unclear as to whether this influenced Mitchell to change his practice.

It is women who nearly always decide on the choice of the family doctor.

It must not be supposed that men are not influenced at all by the things which impress women. The same things do have an effect on them though a weaker one.

Further discussion of the subject, the art of practice, will be in relation to the ideal, as here outlined, and to the special psychology of patients.

The question must now be:-

1. How can the ideal be reached?
2. What are the feelings and impressions that should be aroused and what are the means?
3. How do patients form their judgments?

The answer to the last question is – Through the reason, the aesthetic faculties and through the emotions. Each of these three divisions must be considered separately.

INFLUENCING PATIENTS THROUGH THE REASON

The very important part, complete interrogation and physical examination, has already been given (out of its order). The powerful effect which can be produced by this means is greatly reinforced by:

FULL EQUIPMENT OF DIAGNOSTIC INSTRUMENTS

This will repay itself a hundredfold in the long run. Most patients have been to some other doctor at some time of their lives before coming to you. They will compare your use of diagnostic instruments with what they have before observed. A well equipped outfit gives confidence. It will be reported in a way you hardly suspect, and a strong means of gaining reputation results.

A good Lamp is necessary. If an electric one standing on the desk and connected with the wall plug by a wire is possible, have it. If not a good oil lamp is useful. A frontal mirror is essential. The spectacle frame kind are often uncomfortable. Choose one with an elastic band, or better still, one with a spring over the head which grasps the forehead and occiput. A good one is made by Reynolds and Branson Ltd., Leeds. It is cheap and portable. If you are myopic or young with normal sight, ask for one with a short focal length. If hypermetropic or not young, get one with a long focal length.

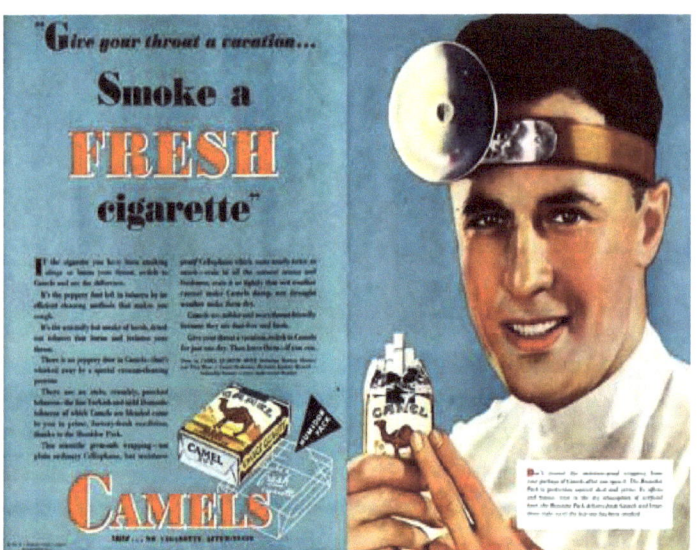

The Medical Tactician

Head mirrors were used to focus a beam of light on to the doctor's area of interest. It became a comic book indication that the wearer was a doctor even to the extreme that a psychiatrist might be using one – presumably peering through to the inner mind!

Throat examinations should always be made with light reflected by the frontal mirror.

A good tongue depressor saves the trouble to the doctor and is less annoying to the patient. Avoid the usual broad hinged variety. Have one with the longest and narrowest blade that your instrument maker keeps, with the handle at right angles.

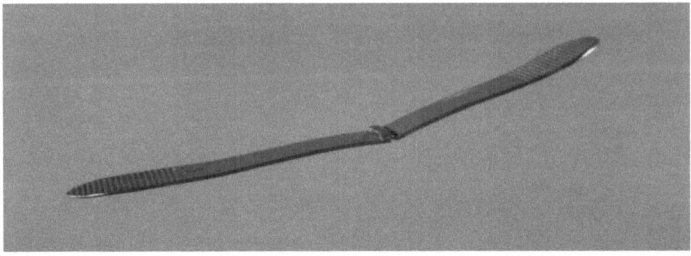

You should have one small laryngoscopic mirror to search for decayed teeth. Use reflected light. Warm the mirror over a flame to prevent condensation of the mouth vapour on it. Before putting in the mouth, test the heat by touching it on the back of your hand.

When visiting, it is well to carry an electric torch for throwing light direct on the throat: they are cheap and portable. When exhausted, the battery can be replaced for a few pence. If not easily obtained locally, write to Gamages Limited, Holborn, London.

Arthur Gamage insisted on selling everything cheaper than anywhere else and would stock everything to do with motoring, cycles, haberdashery and eventually a wide selection of children's toys. He even developed a large mail order business. Quite an entrepreneur of his day.

If you prefer to use a single stethoscope, you should listen afterwards with a binaural, or else the patient thinks you are not up to date or have not heard of everything.

It was 1851 by the time Arthur Leared improved on Rene Laennec's wooden monaural stethoscope by inventing the binaural version. Further advances were made by Cammann in 1852 and it wasn't until the 1940s that the bell and diaphragm model was developed by Rappaport and Sprague.

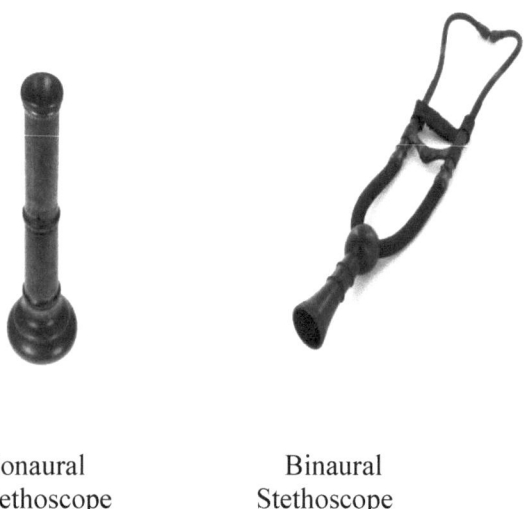

Monaural   Binaural
Stethoscope   Stethoscope

A weighing machine is an excellent thing to have. One weighing machine up to 24 stone can be bought for 21/-. A measuring standard for taking the height of patients, which can be fixed to the wall, can be obtained for 10/6d from Allen and Hanbury, 48, Wigmore Street, London, W.

If weight and height are measured by the doctor the patient feels that more care is taken. To weigh an emaciated child from time to time gives the mother great satisfaction. The confidence resulting well repays the cost of the machine.

A pocket magnifying lens costs 1/6d or 2/-. It is a good plan to inspect all skin diseases with one.

In percussing, use a pleximeter. An ivory one can be had for 2/- or less.

Percussion refers to the art of tapping the tip of the middle finger, held in a curved configuration, against the middle section of the middle finger of the other hand which is pressed firmly and flat against the body part being examined.

It was Leopold Auenbrugger in 1754 who developed the idea of percussion in clinical examination and it is suggested that this idea originated from watching his father tapping kegs to check the level of fluid left. It was Adolph Piorry who ultimately introduced the pleximeter in 1826. It was designed to be placed against the chest and struck with a finger or some other form of percussing instrument. The gradations on the pleximeter were there to act as a reference to the size of the underlying area being defined.

The sound produced by this percussion could be dull and lower pitched suggesting something more solid underneath (try tapping your finger over your kneecap) or could be more resonant and higher pitched as if you were tapping over something less solid such as the air-filled lung.

A level of fluid collection in the chest could be delineated in this way just as Auenbrugger's father would check the level in a keg! The modern clinician finally gave up on the pleximeter and just used the other hand.

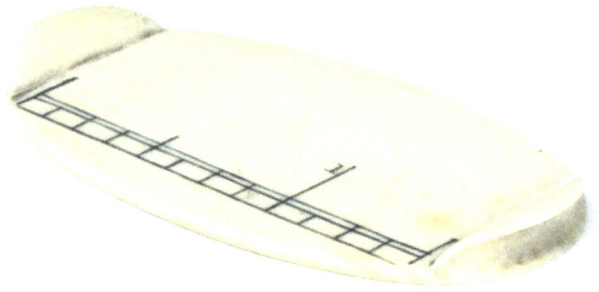

Ivory Pleximeter

A Tucker Wise's cyrtometer for measuring expansive movements of the chest costs 10/6d (Allen & Hanbury), and has a good moral effect on patients anxious about their lungs.

Alfred Thomas Tucker Wise was a physician who specialised in the theory of the curative effects of Swiss altitude in the treatment of tuberculosis. I presume that he developed a chest measuring device to monitor the effects of lung restriction in his patients. He was a house officer at St Mary's Hospital just a few decades before me. He died aged 81 years so his practice in the Swiss Alps may have been beneficial!

A Dermatological pencil for marking the skin when outlining the heart, liver, etc., costs 6d. It helps to convince the patient that a careful diagnosis is being made.

A sphygmograph is valuable; a Dudgeon's costs £2.5.0, or, with Symond's Improved Inkpen for use with plain paper, £2.10.0. The latter obviates the trouble of smoking papers and fixing them. The moral effect is strong and the outlay will repay itself.

Vierordt's sphygmograph was the precursor of the sphygmomanometer and comprised a system of levers hooked to a scale-pan in which weights were placed to determine the amount of external pressure needed to stop blood flow in the radial artery. Not surprisingly, the instrument provided rather imprecise measurements but formed the basic concept for the modern day BP cuff. The Dudgeon's version was probably only used to record pulse rate rather than measuring pressure at the radial artery.

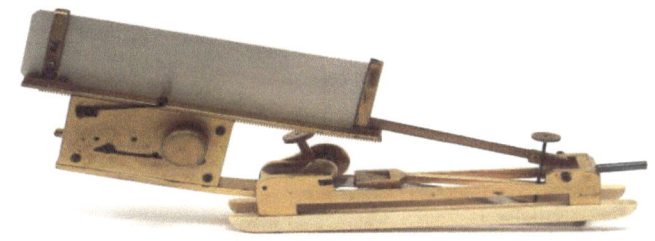

Sphygmograph

It is one of the commonest convictions of patients that their blood is out of order. A profound impression can be made by Haemocytometers and Haemoglobinometers, etc. These are a little costly, but in a good class practice they are well worth having. For directions on how to use them see such work as 'Clinical Methods' by Hutchinson and Rainy.

The Haemocytometer was invented by Louis-Charles Malassez and consists of a thick glass microscope slide with a rectangular indentation that creates a chamber. This chamber is engraved with a grid of perpendicular lines. The area bounded by the lines and the depth of the chamber is known and it is therefore possible to count the number of cells and concentration in a specific volume of fluid.

Have your own diet charts typed and duplicated. Don't use printed ones. You may wish to show patients that you are treating them from your own knowledge.

Temperature charts can be obtained from instrument makers. They should always be used when occasion requires them. Wright & Sons, Ltd., Bristol supply chart holders to fit their own charts. Leatherette 1/-, celluloid 2/-. The metal plate corners, clips and eyelets, give a nice appearance.

If a doctor hangs one of these in the sick room the suggestion is that he is a careful man generally.

If a practitioner has major operations, it looks businesslike to give directions on paper for the preparation. Get them typed. The following may be used as standing or modified.

DIRECTIONS FOR AN OPERATION

Twenty Four Hours Before

Give a saline purgative. If necessary, give copious enema 12 hours before.

A warm bath the day before or morning of the operation, according to circumstances. Use soap freely. If practicable, on the morning of the operation, scrub the part with antiseptic soap. Afterwards cover with a towel wet with Lysol 1%. Over it put a mackintosh.

Dress for Operation

Woollen vest, nightgown and warm stockings, according to the operation

Food

None for 6 hours before.

Immediately before

See that the patient passes urine just before. Remove any artificial teeth.

Preparing the Room

The practitioner should see for himself that the room is suitable. Remove all possible furniture. If the carpet cannot be taken up, cover the floor all round the operating table with clean oil cloth. If necessary, cover the lower part of the window with muslin. Scrub the room and clean it as far as possible two days before. Light a fire the morning of the operation even in warm weather. If a neighbouring room can be used, keep the instruments there till the patient has been anaesthetised. The bed should be warmed with hot water bottles before the operation commences.

Operating Table

If obtainable, this should be 5 or 6 feet long, about 2 feet wide, and from 2 ½ to 3 feet high. If not obtainable, two small tables may be placed end to end. There is no objection to the table being too long if the size of the room permits.

If only short tables can be had, a chair may be placed at one end and the patient's feet rest on this.

Preparation of Instruments

There should be a clean enamelled saucepan ready. The surgeon's instruments should be boiled for 5 minutes with the addition of a little washing soda. A towel should be previously wrapped around the instruments in order that they may be lifted out without touching them with the hand.

One, or better two, small tables for instruments, basins, etc.

Towels   Six

Blankets

Two clean and one clean sheet. One blanket is laid on the table and covered by a sheet. The other blanket covers the patient. Over the sheet lay a clean mackintosh about 3 feet square. Failing this use several clean newspapers.

The Surgeon's Hands

Have ready a nail brush which has recently been boiled, one cake of ordinary soap and one of carbolic soap.

Water

A large ewer of boiling water, another of water which has been boiled and allowed to cool. Keep both covered with towels. The ewers should be cleaned and scalded beforehand. Keep a kettle on the fire.

Dishes

Two basins about a pint size. One large meat dish, two pudding dishes ordinary size.

Receptacle

A slop pail should be placed under the table.

AFTER THE OPERATION

Vomiting

Try sips of soda water, or one drop of Tincture of Iodine in a wineglass of water. If this is ineffective try half-a-teaspoonful of bi-carbonate of soda in 8 tablespoonfuls of warm water. Keep the head of the patient low and a towel round the neck like a child's bib. Heat to the pit of the stomach may be tried.

The Medical Tactician

Hot Bottles

Wrap these well in flannel to prevent burning the feet.

Food

No solid food for 12 hours. If the patient wishes it, tea or well strained coffee may be allowed.

Attendance

Someone should stay in the room till the patient talks coherently. Keep the room dark and well ventilated. Bedpan and urinal may be necessary. A pickle bottle might do as a substitute for one of these.

Visitors

None till the doctor permits. They should not stay too long.

QUESTIONS PATIENTS ARE LIKELY TO ASK

In nearly all cases forgetfulness of the facts of medical science is not in danger of being disclosed, but in instances where it might become evident care should be taken that the requisite knowledge is present. A bad effect is avoided and a good one produced. If asked what is the right weight for a year old baby, an answer must be ready. If lacking, no allowance is made for the difficulty of remembering. A sweeping conclusion follows on the whole knowledge of the practitioner.

It is chiefly in regard to children that awkward questions occur. The following should be committed to memory.-

First Dentition

Central Incisors. - Lower 7th month, upper 8th month.

Lateral Incisors. - Upper 9th month, lower 10th month.

The dates are easy to memorise since they run 7,8,9,10. The order can be recollected by the following means.-

With a pencil place a dot on a piece of paper to represent the supposed position of the lower central incisor. Write '7' near it. Draw a vertical line upwards to reach the supposed position of the upper central incisor. At the end of the line write '8.' From this point draw a line horizontally at right angles to reach the upper lateral incisor. Mark the end with '9.' From this point draw a line vertically downwards to reach the lower lateral incisor. Mark the end of this '10.' A square or parallelogram has been drawn with the lower line missing and '7', '8', '9', '10', at each corner.

The Molars are easy to remember because the first comes at the end of the first year and the second at the end of the second year.

The Canines come midway in time between the Molars, at eighteen months.

Note that at 12 months there should be 12 teeth. Make a point of mentioning that these dates are only an average, that there is irregularity in order and time.

Second Dentition

This is easy to recollect if the molars and Canines are disregarded.

Central Incisors   - 7th year

Lateral Incisors   - 8th year

Anterior Bicuspids   - 9th year

Posterior Bicuspids   - 10th year

The sequence of one tooth a year from before backwards is obvious.

Note that in the case of Central Incisors the Milk Tooth comes at the 7th month and the permanent Incisor at the 7th year.

Molars – The first comes at the 6th year.

The second at the 12th year.

The third at the 18th year – Note the multiples of 6.

The Canines come at the 11th year.

A mnemonic is not easy in this case. The following might be used:-

The letter 'n' is prominent in the word 'canine'. 'n' resembles 11 with the horizontal line left out.

Clinicians and especially medical students have used mnemonics to try and remember the vast lists of associated features in such subjects as anatomy and symptoms. One useful one that I recall is for the causes of chronic intractable cough which is as follows:

GASPS AND COUGH

GORD *(Gastro-oesophageal reflux)*
Asthma
Smoking, Chronic Bronchitis
Post-infection
Sinusitis, post nasal drip
ACE Inhibitor
Neoplasm
Diverticulum
Congestive Cardiac Failure

Outer Ear
***U**pper airway obstruction*
***GI**- Airway fistula*
***H**ypersensitivity*

There are of course many other less tasteful ones such as those referring to the 12 cranial nerves and include, "On old Olympus towering top a fat arsed German ventured a hop".

The Weights of Children

Authorities differ in their figures. The following weights are a means between extremes and have the advantage of being easy to remember:-

At birth the average weight is 7lbs. Mnemonic: The first tooth comes at the 7th month.

At the age of 7 months the weight is doubled to 14lbs.

At the age of 12 months the weight is greater by 12 lbs than at birth. 7 plus 12 = 19lbs or 1 stone 5lbs.

At the age of 2 years add 1 stone to that of the 1st year. 1 stone 5lbs plus 1 stone = 2 stone 5lbs.

At the age of 3 years the increase is comparatively small, 3 lbs, equalling 2 stone 8lbs.

At the 4th year the increase is the same, 3 lbs, equalling 2 stone 11lbs.

In the 5th year the increase is the same, 3 lbs, equalling 3 stone.

At the 10th year the weight is $\frac{10 \text{ stn}}{2}$ = 5 stone.

The above figures are for boys; girls weigh a little less.

At 15 years girls are actually a little heavier and taller than boys. The weight for girls is a little more than $\underline{15 \text{ stn}}$, in
$$2$$
boys slightly less.

At 20 the average weight for men is $\underline{20 \text{ stn}} = 10$ stone
$$2$$
For women it is a little less than 9 stone.

At least this additional pressure has been eased over the years with the excellent research which has produced percentile charts which we all take for granted. You can imagine our conscientious practitioner spending some time remembering all these facts just to avoid being considered not a 'clever man' particularly by his female clients who were most likely to ask such questions. Modern day practitioners can't be expected to know everything about even their own specialty subject. It has been said that specialists know more and more about less and less until they know everything about virtually nothing! A bit harsh perhaps. However, our current doctors will be faced from time to time with patients who have done quite a bit of literature search on the subject of their own condition. They shouldn't be tempted to 'pooh pooh' such presentations as it will only serve (as it did 100 years ago) to make them appear out of date and less reliable. Better to accept the information gracefully, ask for its source and whether it has been critically appraised, with a view to reviewing it and feeding back to them in due course. All part of continuing professional development!

<u>Average Height</u>

These are rarely asked for in young children.

At 10 years boys measure 4 ft. 4 in; girls 4' 3".

At 15 years boys measure 5 ft; girls 5' 1".

At 20 years the average man is 5' 7 ½"; women 5' 3".

Women now cease to grow in height, but men at 24 increase by ½".

The following information is interesting to parents.

In the first five years boys and girls grow equally fast.

From 5 to 10 boys grow faster. From 10 to 15 girls grow faster and at 15 are taller and heavier than boys.

From 15 to 20 males again take the lead.

Failure to Walk

Children usually learn to walk at ages from 12 to 18 months.

Failure may be due to rickets, paralysis, mental deficiency, surgical diseases.

A different case is that where a child has learnt to walk and has 'gone off his legs.' This sometimes occurs in acute illnesses where the child has been laid up and has forgotten his former ability. Assure the mother that walking will come again in time.

Other causes are the incidence of paralysis, rheumatism or surgical diseases.

Other causes would include the various muscular dystrophies, congenital dislocation of the hip and cerebral palsy, all of which may be under his general headings of mental deficiency and surgical diseases.

Failure to Talk

The causes are deafness, mental deficiency. The commonest cause is adenoids

Autism wasn't recognised as a specific condition until 1943 and would have been lumped together under mental deficiency.

INFECTIOUS DISEASES

The incubation period, date of appearance and fading of eruption, period of quarantine and infectiousness, are fully given in Burroughs & Wellcome's Visiting List which is supplied to all practitioners.

To commit the whole table to memory is a formidable task. In some of the diseases it is important that the quarantine after exposure and cessation dates be known. They are likely to be asked at the first visit. There is then no time to look the figures up and an answer must be ready, otherwise a bad impression is created.

These diseases are Diphtheria, Influenza, Measles, Mumps and Whooping Cough.

Some Mnemonics

Varicella ...   Eruption appears on the first day

Scarlatina ...   "   "   "   second day

Small **P**ox ...   "   "   "   third day

Measles   ...   "   "   "   fourth day

Typhus   ...   "   "   "   fifth day

Typhoid   ...   "   "   "   sixth day

Mnemonic - **V**ery **S**ick **P**eople **M**ay **T**ake **T**ea

Eruption of Measles appears on the 4th day. The square of 4 is 16. Quarantine after exposure 16 days. Infectiousness after exposure 16 days. Infection after appearance of rash, 16 days.

Diphtheria begins with a 'D'. Quarantine period after exposure a Dozen days.

Scarlatina has 10 letters. Quarantine after exposure 10 days. It begins with an 'S.' Infectiousness ceases in not less than 6 weeks.

IMPORTANCE OF EXTRA DRUG TREATMENT

The practitioner who confines himself to prescribing a bottle of medicine loses great opportunities of making a strong impression.

The general principle should be to give every possible variety where there is the slightest likelihood of doing any good. This gives the impression that the doctor is 'clever'. Patients know that every doctor can write a prescription or mix a bottle of physic, but they respect a man who shows a wide knowledge of various remedial measures.

In neurasthenics and patients who are nervous about themselves, the more elaborate the instructions are the better; even if the means recommended are of doubtful value. The moral effect in such cases is strong and has a curative power.

Doctors have relied on the placebo effect for centuries and will presumably continue to do so. 'Placebo' is derived from the Latin 'I shall please'. It was first used in the context of an approach to treatment in the latter part of the 18th century and by 1811 it was defined as, 'any medicine adapted more to please than to benefit the patient'. At around the time that our practitioner was writing, Richard Cabot of Harvard medical School is quoted as describing how he "was brought up, as I suppose every physician is, to use placebo, bread pills, water subcutaneously, and other devices." In the excellent historical overview of the placebo effect, by Anton de Craen et al [10], in the Journal of the Royal Society of Medicine, they observe that the value of the placebo was considered to be inversely related to the intelligence of the patient and more effective in the unintelligent, neurotic or inadequate patients. In the same overview they report what may have been the first placebo-controlled trial by John Haygarth in 1801. [11] *At that time a common treatment for many conditions was to apply metallic rods, known as Perkins tractors, to the body. These were supposed to work by electromagnetic influence. He treated 5 patients with placebo tractors made of wood and four of them derived benefit. The next day he obtained identical results with the metal tractors. He notes that "an important lesson in physic is here to be learnt, the wonderful and powerful influence of the passions of the mind upon the state and disorder of the body. This is too often overlooked in the cure of diseases." He concluded that the experiment "clearly proved what wonderful effects the passions of hope and faith, excited by mere imagination was the major mediator between body and mind."*

Without modern day investigations one wonders how many patients succumbed to their underlying diseases during these periods of placebo treatment.

The various means are baths, dietaries, minor operations, special occupation, mental alternatives painful and pleasurable, emotional incentives, imitations, ethical and religious influence, travel, ambition, social influence, climate, dress, special feeding, isolation, varied surroundings, physical and mental shocks, object lessons, commands, study, etc.

The importance of all these varied approaches should not be underestimated and modern medicine has looked at the effects on the immune system of positive/optimistic and negative thought processes. Robert Ader and Nicholas Cohen coined the term 'Psychoneuroimmunology' in1975 [12] *In 1981, they went on to propose that the brain and immune system represent a single, integrated system of defence. Following on from this, in 1985, Candace Pert et al,* [13] *demonstrated that neuro-peptide specific receptors were present on the cell walls of both the brain and immune system which suggested that emotions and immunology are physiologically linked. Most of the research has been biased to the negative effects of stress on immunological defences but research on positive emotional experiences suggests that the opposite may also occur.*

I once saw an elderly gent in outpatients and felt that he probably had a degree of heart failure. I sent him for a chest x-ray with a view to seeing him later in the clinic for further tests. He didn't return and we were worried about him so our staff contacted him to check if he was OK and arrange further review. He said, "That x-ray did me the world of good so I didn't want to bother the doctor anymore."

Every kind of local treatment should be used whenever local treatment is advisable.

These are referred to in detail in the sections on therapeutics.

Here only the general principle is indicated that as many of them should be applied as is possible. Of course care must be taken not to advise expensive things which are likely to be useless, or the effect is very bad.

In this context, the specialty of Allergy comes to mind. Although there are a number of centres of excellence in this field there is a vacuum of expertise in many areas of the UK. This gets filled by practice which is not based on critically appraised science and, in some cases, may well offer relatively expensive interventions which at best don't address the underlying pathology and at worst result in prolonged untreated disease.

Where the patient is well-to-do good is done through the moral influence. Therefore do not hesitate to prescribe for example Digalen, an elegant heart tonic.

Digalen (Hoffmann - La Roche) was a purified Digitalis product which wasn't introduced to the pharmaceutical market until 1904 and once again suggests that our practitioner is writing some time after this date.

At around this time there was some developing tension between the voluntary hospital provision and the private practitioner as exemplified in the following commentary in

'The Hospital – A Journal of the Medical Sciences and Hospital Administration, Vol XLL; No 1,060. Saturday Jan 5th 1907.'

"The question of hospital abuse is one of vital importance to the general practitioner, for by the continual widening of the portals of the hospitals and the free admission to their administrations for all comers, the possible clientele of the private practitioner tends to be proportionately diminished, and his services are increasingly less indispensable to the public. There is also a tendency for the hospitals to move outwards from the Central London district and bring their services to the very doors of the large suburban areas. Again the increased facilities of locomotion by cheap tram services render a visit to a hospital pleasant and inexpensive. There is too in this vast suburban London an ever-increasing unstable proportion of the population, who live in a hand-to-mouth sort of way, have no permanent abode, have no local interests, and make no provision for sickness. They are thrift-less and improvident, yet make a show of respectability and gentility. It is these people who seize every opportunity of getting anything for nothing, who figure conspicuously in the out-patient department of our voluntary hospitals, who support the large suburban theatres and music-halls, but will not support the local doctor so long as a tram-fare will provide them with free medical advice. This free use of the hospitals not only injures the private practitioner by withdrawing from him a large proportion of his clientele in posse, but its moral effect upon the mind of the public is of even greater consequence to him. Instead of the public being taught to estimate their health at a high value, and pay proportionately for its preservation and restoration, this free hospital aid tends to greatly depreciate in their eyes the services of the medical

profession, and accordingly to under-estimate the remuneration such services are entitled to receive. If the present out-patient work of the hospitals were replaced by properly organised provident dispensaries, and if the out-patient department of the hospital were restricted to consultative work, specially sent from these dispensaries or from the private practitioner, the unsatisfactory and cursory examination of the patients by the medical officers of the institution could be ended.

It cannot be gainsaid that the hospital is of infinite service to the private practitioner by supplying, not only a consultant free of charge, but also the technical skill of the specialist and the full equipment of hospital appliances. It is in such cases that the hospital holds its sphere of greatest usefulness, and there can be no better judge of the suitability of a case for hospital treatment than the medical attendant. By a proper restriction of the use of the hospital by the public, a much larger proportion of the community would be compelled to make provision, in one way or another, for the fees of their own doctor, and it would rest with him to decide upon the appropriateness of any particular case for admission to a hospital. Apart from the charitable relief of the suffering, the hospitals have also a great work to perform, both in the education of those entering the profession, and also in the furtherance of medical and scientific knowledge and research. For these purposes the hospitals require material in the sense of the suffering and the diseased. We are of opinion that the hospitals should not suffer from lack of material were they more dependent upon the general practitioner for the selection of cases, whereas the overcrowded condition of the out-patient department might be considerably relieved. This overcrowding consists largely of patients who are of no value to the teacher or the student, but are a considerable burden to the medical officers in charge and a tax upon the financial resources of the hospital. With the increasing difficulties of the general practitioner there is every probability that the number of students entering the profession will continue to diminish, and the unnecessary overcrowding of hospital out-patients, may force itself upon the attention of the hospital authorities by a lack of newly-qualified medical students to offer their free services as medical officers to these departments. There is no doubt that the hospital was never intended to compete with the private practitioner. It should rather be a source of continual assistance and support to him. We shall welcome the day when it can be shown that, by proper provisions and restrictions, the work of the hospital is made supplemental to that of the general practitioner."

The sentiments expressed above are transferrable to the modern day in that some would say that the 'free at the point of delivery' NHS has resulted in a lack of appreciation of this valued service. The abuse of Accident & Emergency departments and failure to attend clinic appointments are just some examples of what can happen if a service is 'free' (apart from National Insurance) with no commitment to payment on the day of treatment.

Voluntary hospitals were independent and relied on local goodwill and other private sources of funding. They were administered by volunteer lay governors and staffed by physicians and surgeons on honorary unpaid contracts. Most of these hospitals began around the mid eighteenth century. The cottage hospitals started appearing around the mid 1800s and were essentially small institutions run by general practitioners in the more rural areas. The long term care of the poor, aged and chronic sick was provided by the Poor Law workhouses and infirmaries. By the 1890s the voluntary hospitals covered around a quarter of all the acute medical care and provided the majority of the medical education.

Some of the hypnotics from Germany are not cheap. The real value is increased by the moral effect of knowing that the price is not small.

There should be good knowledge of patent foods, etc. Most of them have real merit. They are referred to under 'diet'.

The Medical Tactician

Read the advertisements in the medical papers. Write to the proprietors for their printed information and advise them wherever indicated.

In nervous patients inquire in to the daily life. Advise the patient to change his surroundings if these are not good.

The more knowledge you have of treatment other than drugs, the better for the patient and the better for you.

All that you recommend will be talked about and be a legitimate means of gaining reputation.

This finishes what there is to say about influencing patients through the reason. Of course the whole of therapeutics comes under the same heading.

~ CHAPTER 4 ~

INFLUENCING PATIENTS THROUGH THE

AESTHETIC FACULTIES.

- - - - - - - - - - -

Women are much more strongly impressed by this means than men, but on the latter also it has an influence. The effect re-enforces the good impressions made by other means.

THE DOCTOR'S HOUSE.

POSITION:- For general practice the better known the thoroughfare is the better the position. If the street is unfrequented, people will think you are lacking in ambition or that you distrust your own ability or that you have poor judgment. There is a tendency to believe that the best doctors, like the best shops, are to be found in the more public places.

In a back street you are likely to be thought as of timorous, negative material, or lacking in individuality, or in spirit of enterprise and enthusiasm.

The front of the house should be kept in good repair, and well painted. The garden (if any) ought to be as neat and ornamental as possible. The railings (if any) should be well painted.

INFLUENCING PATIENTS THROUGH THE AESTHETIC FACULTIES

Women are much more strongly impressed by this means than men, but on the latter also it has influence. The effect re-enforces the good impressions made by other means.

The Doctor's House

Position: - For general practice the better known the thoroughfare is the better the position. If the street is unfrequented, people will think you are lacking in ambition or that you distrust your own ability or that you have poor judgement. There is a tendency to believe that the best doctors, like the best shops, are to be found in the more public places.

In a back street you are likely to be thought as of timorous, negative material, or lacking in individuality or in spirit of enterprise and enthusiasm.

The front of the house should be kept in good repair, and well painted. The garden (if any) ought to be as neat and ornamental as possible. The railings (if any) should be well painted.

The door should be in the best condition. The door plate ought not be too large and should be kept scrupulously bright. The engraving and block must be good. An old, partly illegible plate signifies failure.

Patients are instinctively attracted or repelled by the outside appearance of a doctor's house. The impressions to be made inside will be helped by those made before entering.

This message rings true when considering the entrances to some of our modern day hospitals (or surgeries). There is nothing worse than the sight of a number of discarded cigarette buts provided by the seriously addicted, who may be sitting in a wheelchair with a drip in situ, just outside the main entrance. The saddest example of this, that I witnessed, was a man who had had an amputation for smoking-related vascular disease and was smoking through a cigarette holder provided by his concerned wife!

If there must be a lamp. Let it be small and in good taste.

A side door for entering is an advantage. If recessed, so much the better. For some reason patients do not like to be seen standing at a doctor's door. See that the bell is answered promptly. If kept waiting, people think the whole house, practitioner included, suffers from slackness.

A cheerful looking servant to answer rings is an acquisition. A sour-faced maid or manservant who looks as if he or she were being troubled, is harmful.

The following is a true anecdote. A lady said to a doctor, "I knew as soon as I saw your man (the footman was a pleasant looking Irishman) I should get well. I went to Sir William - - and the moment I saw his manservant I knew Sir William would never do me any good." Sir William had a particularly funereal looking footman.

For recording messages have the best slate that money can buy. There are slates of white material requiring a lead pencil. Let the latter be tied to the slate.

Do not let members of your family be seen in the hall. This embarrasses patients who think they are intruding.

The waiting room should be light and airy with cheerful pictures on the walls. If the class of practice permits, the drawing room is the best. If a working class practice, let the floor be covered with linoleum. It is well to have varnished wooden walls to a height of 5 feet or so; plain wooden chairs are best.

If there is a special waiting room for patients, light and cheerfulness should be the dominant impression; there should be neither redundancy nor bareness in furnishings. The walls should be light coloured with cheerful pictures.

The Medical Tactician

Back in the 1970s I remember a local GP who was still practising at the age of 90 years! It was clear that his remaining patients had selected themselves out as being survivors and it is doubtful if the various unctions, lotions and syrups that he prescribed for them were doing much good. However, more importantly they weren't doing any harm. He would sit in the middle of his consulting room and the patients would all sit around the edge and were called forward when it was their turn. The occasional button would be undone to examine a limited part of the anatomy. However, we did receive a letter in his spidery hand writing which noted that Joe was the 'champion cigarette smoker of our village and has been coughing more than usual.' He wondered whether he might have lung cancer and was correct! The great advantage the GP has over the Hospital doctor is this longer term knowledge of how individual patients 'tick'. This advantage may be reducing as GPs do less on call and patients see whichever doctor is available on a given day.

If consulting and waiting room adjoin, it is better to have no door between. Patients do not like to go back and face others after a consultation.

This comment reminds me of one of my friends who decided to do a 6 week locum in general practice. He arrived on the Monday morning and the waiting room was heaving with patients. The receptionist settled him in to the small consulting room and then warned him that the first patient was 'a little strange' but not aggressive. He had some vague anal complaint and so my friend asked him to pop on the couch and pull his trousers down so that he could examine him. The room was not only small but badly lit so he pulled over an angle poise lamp, aimed it at his rear end and switched it on. The lamp bulb exploded with a loud bang whereupon the patient leapt to his feet and semi hopped out of the room into the waiting area with his trousers half way up his legs shouting, 'He's not f-----g photographing my arse! 'This had the desired effect of reducing the waiting list by half and the rest of the morning went smoothly.

71

The Medical Tactician

The consulting room should be snug, cosy, and not too large. The general impression to make is that the owner is a man of taste, refinement, learning and NOTHING MORE.

The walls and floor should be well covered. There should not be too much or too little furniture. A desk, a table, a couch and chairs are necessary. These should be the best you can afford. A bookcase as handsome as your means will allow with well bound scientific books, is desirable.

Every instrument of diagnosis that you can afford should be in evidence. A microscope, ophthalmoscope, frontal mirror, stethoscope, test tube stand, spirit lamp, and reagents may lie on the table. The medical journals may be there also.

The walls may be decorated with good etchings, engravings and photographs of professional friends and teachers.

A gallery of portraits of medical celebrities looks well.

Flowers and busts are in good taste. On the mantelpiece a non-striking clock is best.

Do not display political or religious emblems. Don't let even a newspaper be seen.

All other instruments but those of diagnosis should be kept out of sight. Catheters, splints, bandages etc. must not be seen. Bones, skulls, anatomical plates, etc. are in the worst taste.

It is needless to say there should be no pipe rack or ash trays in view.

While everything should point to the owner as an earnest, enthusiastic, and scientific professional man, there should be NOTHING MORE.

If you have any hobbies, keep them out of the patient's sight. Don't exhibit stuffed birds, pinned butterflies, pickled specimens, etc.

We have known a man who kept snakes bottled in spirit under the impression that they gave his consulting room a scientific look.

Let your billheads be neat and your notepaper good, with the address embossed.

In brief, let your house give the impression you are an enthusiastic, scientific, and cultivated man who is methodical and has no hobbies. Let nothing else be suggested HOWEVER INNOCENT IT MAY BE.

All your patients, and women especially, will estimate you by what they see and by what they do not see.

If you dispense, the dispensary is much better out of sight of patients.

If this is impossible, then the bottles, jars, etc. must be numerous and as good as those of a first class chemist's shop.

Have your labels neatly printed. Messrs. Suttley and Silverlock, Blackfriars Road, London, produced the first of the following two:-

Shake the Bottle

The Mixture

From Dr Smith

Compare it with the common one below.

_____

_____

It is advisable to have "Shake the Bottle" on all labels.

In a town where there are several chemists it will be found that there is one doing most of the trade. His shop is very likely the cleanest and handsomest. He dispenses prescriptions in bottles of the best glass with good corks, which are neatly capped. The label is well engraved and the wrapper artistically done up.

Why does he take extra trouble with a little extra cost? He knows human nature. He knows the public judge by appearances, that they will estimate the quality of his drugs by the get-up of his bottles. He knows that attention to these details pays. He knows he has competitors and that if he takes less care than they he will be compared unfavourably with them.

There is more than one business firm in London that uses an artistic paper for doing up packages and a special tape for tying them. They show by this means respect for their goods and this respect radiates to the customer.

A well known business man has said he would rather try to sell inferior goods in a good package than better ones in a bad package.

Why are medical men so often indifferent to the packages in which they dispense drugs? Because firstly, they have not got the business instinct developed. Secondly, they have got in to a groove and know that their competitors are equally careless. Thirdly, they do not realise the good advertisement they are missing. They do not realise how their patients judge them by such small matters. Fourthly, they unconsciously feel that there are other factors of more importance and think that these swamp details of this kind. It is a mistake to think that such details are swamped. They are noticed and talked about.

If things of this kind are important in business where the goods speak, how much more important must they be in medical practice where the patients frequently have to and do judge by appearances alone?

The following is an instructive case. A certain student had great difficulty in passing his examinations. He eventually succeeded in qualifying. His medical knowledge was limited but he was well qualified in a knowledge of human nature. He started in practice with a very small nucleus. He attended to every trifling detail and was soon doing a practice £1,000 a year.

THE DOCTOR'S PERSON

A strong impression is conveyed by clothes. They indicate the respect a man has for himself and for others. With them are associated the ideas of success or of failure according as they are good or otherwise.

Let your hat be irreproachable, your collars and cuffs immaculate, your clothes of good material and fashionably cut, your boots well polished and with no signs of wear.

Your hair should never be untidy; your face should be cleanly shaved or your beard neatly trimmed. Your finger nails ought not to be in mourning; your hands should be white and out-of-doors covered with well fitting gloves.

The Medical Tactician

The sun tan was not fashionable then. In fact any indication that one had been exposed on a daily basis to the sun's rays suggested that one was of a lower social class and had, of necessity, to work out doors. At the end of the 19th century the upper classes wore plenty of clothing protection to avoid getting sun tanned and the parasol was a popular accessory for women.

If you wished to place your son in a school, you would be influenced by the recommendations of other parents and by the success of the pupils in passing examinations. If possible you would visit the school. If you found it well appointed and the proprietor unimpeachably dressed, the confidence inspired by the recommendations would be confirmed. If the schoolmaster were a wise man he would leave you under this impression and do nothing to let you think that he was not giving his whole time and thought to the important subject of education. He would be well advised to keep any hobbies out of sight, not to show you the dogs with which he went ratting or the invention at which he had been working hard for the last year, or his intimate acquaintance with latest novels. If he were careless in his dress or if the house and school appointments were not good you would go away with a shaken confidence.

Important as such things are to a schoolmaster, they are still more so to a doctor. Microscopic eyes inspect every detail of your practice and of your house. Your notepaper is noted, your medicine packages are criticised, and by all these things you are judged.

Unfounded as are such data for estimating your professional skill, it is nevertheless on them that you are largely appraised.

In all these details you can get a perfectly legitimate advertisement which pays for itself, which may yield a dividend of 1,000 per cent or more in the year.

The Medical Tactician

The impressions made through the eyes are never disclosed to you but they are disclosed to friends and at tea parties in a way of which you may have no conception.

Dress should convey that you are a highly cultivated man and NOTHING MORE. Avoid glaring ties, a heavy watch chain, perfumery, or any sign that you are a dandy. The impression would follow that you wished to make an impression, that you are not satisfied with your real good qualities. The effect is something akin to that of a man who boasts; there is a feeling of reaction against him.

If you have a motor or a carriage, don't have a cheap one; it is better to wait till you can afford one with a good appearance. Otherwise you are giving yourself an advertisement that is bad.

I am reminded of my first request, as a new Consultant, to see a patient referral in a neighbouring hospital. I was still driving a rather battered old car and unfortunately the day of the referral the exhaust finally gave up. I drove in to the Consultants' car park (they had them in those days) with a throaty roar from my rear (i.e. the car's). A horrified jobsworth with a peaked cap rushed over to prevent me from maneuvering my wreck in to place. It was only after waving my stethoscope at him and providing ID that he let me park!

More than once in the above remarks the words "NOTHING MORE" occur in capitals. Under the heading of "INTERVIEW" the injunction is given that after the prescription stage conversation should be limited, that the doctor should only say enough to avoid appearing unsociable and NOTHING MORE. The psychological reason is that when the desired impressions are made, these remain much stronger if there is NOTHING MORE conveyed, however innocent.

In a portrait the artist refrains from putting in any detail such as a background with the scenery since these would only weaken the effect.

It is to your interest to make the strongest impression possible and do nothing to lessen it. The psychology of the "NOTHING MORE" rule will be referred to again.

INFLUENCING PATIENTS THROUGH THE EMOTIONS

Some overlapping in treating the whole subject of the art of practice is unavoidable, because the factors themselves overlap.

For example, confidence is produced by both emotion and reason. A cock-sure manner acts through the emotions, a systematic physical examination acts through the intelligence; both combine to one effect. The two in this case reinforce one another.

Under the heading of 'The Ideal' various qualities were mentioned as contributing to the patient's confidence that she is in good hands. The more numerous the impressions leading to one effect the stronger and more lasting this is.

Therefore the importance of arousing every feeling in your favour which is possible becomes obvious.

The emotions are strong moving forces. A patient with confidence in your ability and no other special feeling may recommend you. But if confidence is combined with gratitude she is much more likely to talk about you and probably with extravagant praise.

The emotions which can be aroused are

1.   Respect

2.   Admiration for professional ability

3.   Gratitude

If a new patient called on a practitioner and found his house and personal appearance corresponding to that recommended in previous pages, there would be intellectual belief that she had probably come to a competent man. But there would be more than an intellectual belief. There would be a feeling of respect before a word was spoken. There would follow the impression that the medical man had respect for himself and for others. This emotional condition can be greatly strengthened - or it can be destroyed.

At the reception and dismissal of a patient there is a non-professional relation. The greeting and the goodbye form part of the ordinary social intercourse. The heartiness of manner must be proportionate to the intimacy of the acquaintanceship. The impression to be conveyed is that you are a strong man, who feels secure in his position, who is courteous and kind as a strong man can afford to be, who is pleased to see the patient, not because of the fee but from natural amiability and professional interest.

Our practitioner puts his finger on one of the very basic and often tricky aspects of the doctor-patient relationship. How do we approach the basic social interaction with our patients? It very much depends on the circumstances and the individual that we are dealing with. As a very junior doctor I once said to an elderly female patient, "How are we today my dear?" She stared at me over some half moon glasses for a moment and then said, "I've no idea how you are and I'm certainly not your dear!" I never made that mistake again but I suspect such a question might not have produced such a sharp response from another elderly lady.

The use of the first name instead of the surname is also a contentious issue. Nursing staff have become much more sensitive to individuals' preferences as to how they wish to be addressed. Most will ask the patient what their preference is and will often find that the first name appearing on their record, although being the official one, has been hated since birth and it is the middle or nickname that should be used.

One of our receptionists in outpatients let me know, with a wry smile, that one of the patients that morning, when referring to me, had said something to the effect that Steve had wanted to see him again as his case was getting more complicated. Such comments should sound a large warning bell in the back of the mind and any reciprocation of familiarity will be seized upon by the individual as a sign that the doctor has a special regard for him or her and will provide preferential treatment.

We are all human of course and some patients by nature of their bon hommie, wit, stoicism in adversity and selflessness will stand out. After prolonged periods of care, it may feel natural to call them by their first names but interestingly it is less common for the patient in these circumstances to prefer to call the doctor by their first name; often preferring to stick with 'doctor'. General Practitioners, as opposed to secondary care physicians, may well have looked after a particular patient for decades, since childhood, and in such circumstances may be both on first name terms.

The much more serious aspect of the doctor-patient relationship is of course the implication that the relationship is more than strictly professional. One of my colleagues (when we were much younger) saw a female patient of about the same age, in outpatients, a couple of times. From his point of view these were straight forward and unremarkable consultations but a short time later the patient turned up at his house. He was at work and his wife opened the door to be confronted by this woman who proceeded to profess her undying love for my colleague!

The man with the ways of an obsequious tradesman or a dancing-master, who is oily-tongued and says "Well, and how are we to-day?" is seen through and despised.

With social superiors (if that is possible), social equals and those just a little lower in the social scale, politeness must never be overdone.

With working people a greater heartiness in the tone of voice is desirable, while avoiding any undignified familiarity. Such patients are often embarrassed at meeting their "betters," afraid that they are giving trouble or intruding. An enforced geniality is not resented even if seen through. It is gratefully accepted as meaning a desire to put them at their ease.

Pompousness is not a sign of strength and will not be so recognised. If exhibited in the consulting-room it is resented, leads to under-estimation of really good qualities and will be related with ridicule to others.

The same remark applies to conceit, vanity, artificiality, affectation. All these things are as transparent in a medical man as in anybody else.

Solemnity has some resemblance to pompousness; it is the negative of cheerfulness. The successful man is not likely to be solemn, and the quality will be likely to be considered as a sign of want of success.

Like cheerfulness, solemnity is contagious, and an unpleasant state of mind is produced.

The Medical Tactician

The man with the ways of an obsequious tradesman or a dancing-master, who is oily-tongued and says "Well, and how are we today?" is seen through and despised.

With social superiors (if that is possible), social equals and those just a little lower in the social scale, politeness must never be overdone.

With working people a greater heartiness in the tone of voice is desirable, while avoiding any undignified familiarity. Such patients are often embarrassed at meeting their 'betters', afraid that they are giving trouble or intruding. An enforced geniality is not resented even if seen through. It is gratefully accepted as meaning a desire to put them at their ease.

Pompousness is not a sign of strength and will not be so recognised. If exhibited in the consulting-room it is resented, leads to under-estimation of really good qualities and will be related with ridicule to others.

The same remark applies to conceit, vanity, artificiality, affectation. All these things are as transparent in a medical man as in anybody else.

Solemnity has some resemblance to pompousness; it is the negative of cheerfulness. The successful man is not likely to be solemn, and the quality will be likely to be considered as a sign of want of success.

Like cheerfulness, solemnity is contagious, and an unpleasant state of mind is produced.

The bad effect of depression is too obvious to require comment. If this unfortunately exists it should be counteracted by an enforced cheerfulness.

It is unnecessary to say that ill-temper is fatal.

It has already been mentioned that patients, women especially, pay more attention to the tone of voice than to the words spoken. Therefore every statement of diagnosis and treatment should be made in a tone of conviction.

A man who is confident by nature can do this easily. The man who is not can cultivate the ability. Such a one should first think to himself the reason for what he pronounces and state his belief with all the earnestness which such conviction gives.

It is better to be sure, cocksure, even if occasionally mistakes are made, than to go through life expressing doubt. Mistakes will do harm but much less harm than a hesitating manner. Patients want a doctor who is cocksure.

It is interesting to note our practitioner's use of the word 'cocksure' as this would imply a certain arrogant overconfidence and I suspect could also be a turn-off for the average patient. There is no doubt that super confidence can be very reassuring to a patient and, provided that the doctor has sound medical knowledge, may enhance the whole doctor-patient relationship. However, the higher one's esteem reaches with the patient the greater the fall when a mistake occurs.

A doubtful diagnosis can be given in an emphatic manner. For example, a child appears to be sickening for something, perhaps an eruptive fever. You can say as if you were certain, as if every medical man would be certain, that the exact nature can only be told by further observation. You know this is true, therefore let it be said with all the assurance which this knowledge gives.

Whooping cough is prevalent. A child is suspected but has not yet whooped. State emphatically that there are no means of distinguishing whooping cough till the special sound is heard. The emphasis will show that the doubt is inherent in the circumstances and does not depend on faulty diagnostic power.

The impressions of earnestness, candour, naturalness and simplicity will follow easily if the practitioner gives his undivided attention to the case, rigidly excluding everything else from the mind; and if he is systematic and thorough, formulating definitely to himself the diagnosis and treatment and then gives these clearly to the patient and does NOTHING MORE.

When a doctor has done those things which he ought to do he has attained the maximum effect. He can only weaken it by further talk.

A certain lady in London was asked if her dentist were a good one. She answered, "Yes, a very good dentist, but he is a bounder; he will talk about his motor cars".

This man was lessening the good effect he produced by neglecting the NOTHING MORE rule.

A practitioner's consulting room, his whole tone and manner ALONE should give the impression he is earnest and studious.

If he mentions that he sits up late at night studying, the indirect attempt to produce an effect is seen through. We have known a doctor say this and it cost him a patient who was shrewd.

It is unwise to mention the titled people you have just been to see or even when asked to say you are busy. It is better to reply that you are satisfied.

Above all, keep your private amusements and hobbies out of sight, however innocent they may be.

ADMIRATION FOR PROFESSIONAL SKILL

This is primarily a judgment not an emotion. But when the impression is very strong it passes into the emotional stage. Then it becomes an excellent advertising force.

It induces the patient to talk about her doctor with praise and often with extravagant words, when if merely satisfied and nothing more she would not talk of him at all.

It is produced by the means described under the headings of Interview, of Routine and lastly by a thorough knowledge of extra-drug treatment.

It should be remembered that most patients have sooner or later consulted more than one medical man and often for the same complaint. They have had opportunities of comparing one with another. It is also true that many practitioners are decidedly weak in therapeutics outside text book treatment. The man who can bring the heaviest battery of remedial measures to bear scores simply by comparison with his competitors.

An impression of knowledge and skill is strongly conveyed, but this is not all. Little tips that give comfort, details of nursing, full instructions in diet, a thousand and one means other than drugs which can be used become the subject of gossip and are a powerful advertisement.

To give one example. A patient was under treatment some months for an ulcer of the leg. He then consulted another medical man who applied a Martin's bandage. The ulcer healed in three weeks. Here the success was a subject of conversation, but in addition the means used stimulated talk.

Henry Martin 1824–1884 was the first to use a wide, rubber, roller bandage to treat vascular ulcers.

Whenever a good impression of skill is made, this is magnified if the emotional conditions have also been brought about, and the advertising force is much stronger.

If on the other hand the practitioner is not respected or is somewhat disliked, the tendency is to minimise his ability.

When recommending a remedy it is not a good plan to say to the patient anything like the following:-

"I used this treatment lately with very good results." It implies that your experience in this respect is limited, or may be limited.

Use no words that might signify the measure is new or that you have only employed it lately.

AROUSING A PATIENT'S GRATITUDE

This is one of the most valuable feelings to bring about. It is produced by courtesy, carefulness, sympathy, the belief that you are doing your best, etc.

In addition to such means which can be generalised there are numerous ways which cannot be generalised. These depend on the particular conditions. For example; sending a special messenger with medicine in a distressing case or visiting her early in the morning.

There are a thousand and one means of accomplishing the object which arise out of the circumstances.

The golden rule is, put yourself in the patient's place and think of everything that could add to her comfort or her welfare.

~ CHAPTER 5 ~

<u>TACT</u>

An assistant was discharged from a shop for forgetting the name of the customer. A newspaper, hearing of the case, interviewed the manager of a large department store, and asked him for comments on it. His remarks were published as follows:-

"Nothing annoys customers more, especially ladies, than to be asked for their name and address, if they are very often in the shop. I suppose it flatters them a little to be recognised. We should none of us like to feel that we are so ordinary as to leave no impression on people. Now in such a case as this one I dare say it might just turn the scale in favour of making an occasional customer into a regular one if the assistant had said 'Thank you, Madam' and murmured the address to show he had recollected it. Then the customer would go away thinking 'very attentive they are in this shop. Pleasant young man that'. And the fish is caught. Whereas if she is asked for name and address just as if she had never been in the shop before, she feels like an outsider. The whole secret of success in our business lies in the cultivation of a sense of intimacy between customer and shop. We actually lost a customer the other day because I did not recognise her voice on the telephone. 'Surely you know me by this time' she said. 'I have dealt with you long enough'. She did not deal with us any more though".

If it is necessary for a tradesman to make a customer think he takes a personal interest in her, much more is it necessary for a doctor to do this with his patient.

Every individual must be made to think that she is the most favoured patient or at least that there is no one more favoured.

This applies no matter what the social status may be.

The Medical Tactician

A medical man visiting a well-to-do patient saw a servant who was under his treatment and said to her, "You need not come for the medicine, I will bring it tomorrow if I don't forget."

Though he did not forget, his thoughtless remark cost him the patient. It implied that he did not consider her of first importance and might not remember.

A rule to keep in mind is that patients do not make allowances.

A busy man has his memory greatly taxed, but no excuses will be made for him on these grounds.

To forget to put up a bottle of medicine or anything else promised is likely to cause resentment, to lead to the loss of a patient and to ill-natured remarks.

The following is a case in point.

A practitioner promised to get a special drug. He forgot it. He lost the patient, the patient's friends, and some of his good reputation.

Never trust to memory. Carry a notebook. Put down everything and leave nothing to chance.

Our practitioner makes no mention of any secretarial support and I can only infer that he performed all his own administrative tasks himself. Most modern day doctors rely heavily on their secretaries and consider them an essential part of the medical team. A personal secretary who makes sure that important results of investigations are brought to your attention, copes with patient enquiries but knows when to involve you, knows your working week and how to gauge whether to interrupt you at any point in time, types letters that don't need constant proof reading and reminds you about important correspondence that is pending, is worth her/his weight in gold.

This becomes painfully apparent if for any reason there is an abrupt change in secretarial support and you have to rely on a substitute temporary secretary who, for no fault of their own is much less experienced. One of my Gynae colleagues, who had become confident in the accuracy of his secretary's letters, while rushing to another commitment, made the mistake of not checking an agency letter and this was returned by the GP with the following single letter underlined:

"This unfortunate lady has been suffering with vaginal thrust for the last 3 years." Easily done when you see how close the 't' and 'h' are on the keyboard!

The guidance nowadays is that a copy of all correspondence is sent to the patient. This is a very worthy principle but adds an extra pressure on the doctor, in that dictation will need to be couched much more in lay terms and secretaries are more likely to get regular phone calls asking for clarification of particular terms within the letter.

It is much easier to fall than to rise.

If you meet a patient in the street whom you have not seen for some time, inquire genially how he is, to show that you take an interest in him. If the family are the patients, don't forget to make a similar inquiry.

I was once approached in the local shopping centre by a lady who grasped me by the arm and with a very earnest tone said to me, "Dr Connellan, David died." Unfortunately, I didn't recognise her with any confidence and there had been a number of Davids under my care in the previous year, not all of whom had died, I might add. I managed to collect myself and, hoping not to offend, responded with equal gravitas, "I'm so sorry to hear that. How have the family taken it?" I'm sorry to say that I never did find out which particular David was being referred to.

Many people when consulting a doctor for slight ailments feel a little ashamed to do so.

He will think he will laugh at them for coming over trifles. They often apologize for giving trouble.

Never omit to reassure them that they are quite wise to have advice, that it is important to attend to little things.

Keep your tongue-depressor where the patient can see it is in a clean place, and after using it put it in a basin or somewhere that will show it is put away to be washed, and that there is no danger of your thinking it is now clean.

A dentist who enjoyed a large practice made it an invariable rule to wash his hands in the presence of the patient before examining the mouth. He had tact in this. The fact was not only noted but also commented on. A little thing like this was an excellent advertisement. Therefore before touching the mucous membrane of the mouth, wash your hands in the consulting room, or if that is not possible leave the room to do so and mention the reason. Do this even if you know your hands are clean.

Hand hygiene has, quite rightly, become a major issue within the medical profession, particularly in light of the prevalence of multi-resistant bacteria in health professional environments. Patients are advised to observe their doctors/nurses and check that they have washed their hands or used alcohol gel before and after examining them. Such essential hygiene will inevitably lengthen the average ward round if the doctor has to see and examine 30 patients in one round.

The irony is that later that day a nurse may well do a trolley round checking vital signs using the same blood pressure cuff and oximeter finger clip on consecutive patients. There is the additional risk that patients' visitors will enter the ward without any hand hygiene and be inadvertent carriers of such bacteria.

In suitable cases give a dose of medicine with your own hand, and if circumstances warrant it, stay to see the effect.

When you are told of what has been done by the patient himself or others before you were consulted, do not pooh-pooh it and smile a sarcastic smile even if you do not agree with the remedy. Give credit to well-meant efforts and you will enhance your reputation for kindness and sympathy.

Do not be obstinate in opposing suggestions by nurses and friends if they are good ones. Listen patiently to every sensible proposal. It may be wise to allow it for the mental effect. Be frank in giving credit to any good idea. If you oppose a suggestion let it be clear that you do it from conviction and not from any obstinacy. But take care that all your advice is as complete as possible. Leave as little room as you can for suggestions to come from others. You must yourself think of everything that can be done. If obvious things are suggested, you have failed in care. Be careful about your explanations of what is the matter. It is extraordinary how the statements of a doctor can be distorted. Be on your guard especially with unintelligent people. While it was advised that the rationale of therapeutics should not be given, this does not apply to explanations of the disease present. A pencil sketch or diagram illustrating points that are not clear give great satisfaction and make people think you understand the subject. If you possess fluency of speech and can illustrate your points by apt comparisons, make use of this ability. But if you are not good at speaking do not talk more than is necessary. In any case beware of not making your meaning plain. To fail in this respect gives a bad impression. Therefore do not attempt an explanation where the apprehension is doubtful. Be slow, very slow to confess, or even allow the inference that you are puzzled or have reached the limit of your resources. School your face not to show your doubts. Your every expression is watched with microscopic eyes.

Occasionally a patient thinks he knows more than the doctor about his illness. In such a case make the examination as complete as possible. Do not enter into any discussion. After the first visit, shorten the length and number of visits as much as you can. Only say what is absolutely necessary.

Give your directions in a short and decisive manner and allow no discussion.

In acute cases make it a rule not to give or prescribe large quantities of medicine where the remedy may have to be changed. If you have given a prescription people will complain of the cost and if you dispense yourself the unnecessary medicine will suggest want of foresight.

With the explosion of drug therapies and medical/surgical interventions, the cost of health care is a worldwide concern which has led to 'post code lotteries', explicit rationing of health care and 'market place' style competition between providers at a time when patients are increasingly aware of the range of therapeutic options potentially available to them. This is an inevitable source of tension between governments, health professionals and patients.

Unused bottles of medicine impair confidence.

Do not order expensive instruments which may not prove a success. The failure might be associated with the idea of incompetence on your part.

Avoid nauseous mixtures as far as possible.

To prescribe drachm doses of Tincture of Chiretta is unpardonable.

Chiretta, or chirayta, consists of the dried plant, Swertia Chirata, an annual herb, indigenous to the mountainous districts of Northern India. The drug consists chiefly of the stem, which is of a dark purplish-brown colour. It may be distinguished by its colour, intensely bitter taste, and continuous pith.

Chiretta owes its action to its bitterness; it is used in dyspepsia to improve the appetite. It is usually administered in the form of infusion.

I assume that our practitioner was concerned to avoid such high doses of this bitter concoction.

If it is really necessary to give unpalatable drugs, warn the patient and say it is unavoidable.

Handle highly nervous people, those with sensitive skins, with delicate palates or treacherous stomachs, with deliberate care; remember that operations which fail or disagreeable medicines which are unsuccessful are likely to injure your reputation or even cause your dismissal. Therefore give hypochondriacs who are fond of attention but not of drugs, tasteless or palatable medicine.

Unless there is a real need, do not ask a patient to take medicine before breakfast, or during the night.

Always use poison bottles for poison, or at least a printed label with these words on

"Not to be taken"

To do otherwise is to show you are not a careful man.

Do not get a reputation for heroic remedies.

The high colour of the urine in people whose skin is active may cause alarm. Explain the relation between the skin and the kidneys.

When telling a patient he may take anything he likes, say "anything simple". Then if he takes sausages or anything which disagrees you can retort that you said anything simple.

If you give a medicine labelled 'Every 4 hours', do not forget to say whether the patient is to be awakened from sleep or not.

If the directions are in spoonfuls, remember that spoons vary in size.

If you dispense, have your bottle graduated.

Do not take your wife with you on your rounds. People think she is likely to ask what is the matter and that you will tell her. Do not let your wife or relatives boast about your skill, your successful cures, etc. It will be thought this is an attempt to bring grist to the mill.

Do not turn a case over to a specialist unless there is a real need. But do not fail to do so if it is necessary.

Avoid the following mistake which was actually made. A medical man treated a case of lachrymal obstruction with a lotion when it was hopeless to expect this means to succeed.

The patient on her own initiative consulted a specialist, learnt the truth, and the story became current with considerable damage to the attendant's practice. Make a study of remembering all that was said or done at each visit. To forget the instructions you gave creates the impression that you have little interest in the case or that you have a bad memory, either entails loss of confidence.

Make notes. Carry a notebook and put down everything. This means extra trouble but it well repays itself.

A knowledge of shorthand is very valuable to medical men. To those who do not know any system and have the enterprise to learn one, Gregg's can be strongly recommended. (Publisher, W.S. Partridge, London).

It can be learnt in 80 hours - about one-tenth of the time required by the popular systems, and it is equally good. By those who think such an undertaking too much, a contracted long hand can be easily prepared.

The number of words descriptive of patients' conditions is limited. Prominent consonants suggest the whole word. For example, "pn" may stand for pain, "ap" for appetite, "tng" for tongue, etc.

The Medical Tactician

Over the last century, doctors have developed a shorthand 'language' to facilitate history taking, particularly when faced with large numbers of patients needing to be assessed in diminishing and valuable time. The following passage, although somewhat of a caricature, provides a flavour of what is possible:

This 88 year old ♀ C/O SOBOE, PND and more recent chest tightness and SOA. She has a PMH of DM, AF and mild LVF. O/E her BP150/85, p irreg 82/min. HS revealed mod MR and there was B/L pitting SOA. There were bibasal fine insp crackles. No clinical evidence of DVT. She appears to have developed CCF on a background of MVD and AF. Current Rx comprises Gliclazide 40mg od, Furosemide 40mg od, Dig 0.125mg od, Enalapril 2.5mg od, Warfarin (to reduce the risk of CVA) and Ibuprofen 400mg prn (for LBP). The latter +ACEI + NSAID puts her at risk of renal dysfunction so we will be checking U&Es before any change of Rx. Also FBC, LFTs and Trop T. Please note the DNAR request, by her, on her last admission.

There has also developed a less respectful number of slang acronyms. Medical practitioners, in keeping with all human beings, may from time to time feel frustrated by their patients for a variety of reasons and some will obtain relief by resorting to black humour or 'amusing' acronyms which they feel summarise the case or situation in times of stress. Some examples include:

4F – Fat, fortyish, flatulent, female – all of which may indicate a higher risk of gall bladder disease.

Ash cash – Doctor's fee for signing a cremation form

Granny dumping (or Pop Drop) – Delivering elderly relative to A&E and then disappearing.

Frequent flyer - Someone who is transported to and from hospital on a routine basis (also someone who spends more time at the local hospital than most employees and is known by all staff members including Social Services)

LOBNH – Lights on but nobody home

Brothel Sprouts – Genital warts

Lipstick sign – If a female patient is well enough to apply it, she is well enough to be discharged from hospital.

The O sign – Patient comatosed with mouth open – may be followed by the Q sign when the tongue starts protruding and death may be imminent.

TATT – Tired all the time

TEETH – Tried everything else try homeopathy.

TFBUNDY – This is one of the more shocking ones which seems at first to be seriously callous and uncaring but may summarise the feeling of the medical team in a desperate situation which is felt to be irretrievable. 'Totally f----d but unfortunately not dead yet'. Not to be recommended and probably not used anymore but a good example of one of the extreme doctor slang acronyms.

At a visit it is better as a rule to give chief attention to the reports and remarks of the head of the family, if he is present, and address your opinions and explanations to him. If you do not do this, the sensitive "head one" may think himself slighted.

How much to tell a patient may sometime be a nice point. A good rule to follow is to tell him as much as is good for him to know. It may be good for him to know anything simple which is within his comprehension. It is not good for him to know the rationale of treatment.

The approach to patient information has of course dramatically changed over the last few decades and informed consent has become de rigueur. The paternalistic approach adopted by our practitioner would not be tolerated in today's medical management. Knowing the full facts about any intervention or treatment and the risks *entailed, down to the severe <1% variety and death rate, will inevitably induce a bit more patient stress and also make the decision as to whether to proceed more difficult. However, clinicians have become much more litigation aware and their defence unions would be uncomfortable if the providers of such treatment were economical with the full facts. The complexity of modern medicine makes it much more imperative to be up front with our patients even if this dialogue is more fraught than the old comment, 'Let me worry about that'.*

I do wonder how we would cope if such an approach was taken up by e.g. airlines. We would receive an information sheet, with our booking, informing us of the risks which might include acute tobacco withdrawal, circulating viruses, TB, peanut allergen, relative oxygen desaturation, pilot error, lengthy transfer time to nearest hospital, turbulence damage, sleep deprivation, DVT /PE and death!

NURSES

Use tact and discernment in your attitude to nurses and attendants on the sick. A nurse can do much harm or good. Their statements weigh with patients and the public. Take a nurse to some extent into your confidence. Remember they are very sensitive to blame or praise. If you have to disagree with a nurse over some matter, do so tactfully, not to throw discredit on her skill or judgment. Make a point of praising her efforts when you can. To do so naturally is very likely to make her your friend.

Doctors nowadays rely a great deal on their nursing colleagues and indeed on what have become known as Allied Healthcare Professionals (which include physiotherapists and occupational therapists). The multidisciplinary team approach has been the 'buzz' target in recent years and the patient is the central focus of that team, whether it be the Consultant-led ward based team, GP practice with practice nurses or the specialty-based multidisciplinary team (MDT) e.g. in cancer care.

The Medical Tactician

The senior nurse on a ward is likely to know more about protocols of care than the fledgling junior doctor dealing with the day to day management.

There will always be individual examples of both poor nursing and doctoring but team work will usually help to iron out such imperfections in the best interests of the patient. Our practitioner will have been faced with a team of possibly just two with all the potential tensions that might arise from such a situation, particularly when the patient was deteriorating.

When attending a primipara, explain that the lump in the hypogastrium is normal. Otherwise it may cause alarm.

When giving an anaesthetic to a nervous patient, continue to ask if he feels an itching at the nose. His attention is attracted to this expected symptom which never comes and his nervousness is lessened.

Preaching to immoral patients seldom does any good. It is better to appeal to the sense of self-preservation.

When examining a patient, don't say "This looks strange" or "That is curious".

Avoid saying, "I think the disease is so-and-so". Say positively that it is -- what you think it is. If you have made a mistake in diagnosis or treatment, do not be too ready to admit it. Say nothing.

With neurasthenic and hysterical cases do not say there is nothing the matter. Even the friends may not believe you. Assure them that you understand the suffering, that the symptoms will pass away and that the patient will get well. Treat the case with as much apparent seriousness as if it were severe.

It is tempting to speculate that our practitioner might have been inclined to fall back on the diagnosis of neurasthenia more frequently than today's equivalent and this wouldn't

98

be surprising as the investigative armamentarium was much more limited. How many cases of e.g. thyrotoxicosis may have been given this label? However, some doctors are much better than others in sorting out the 'wheat from the chaff'. Those that are less gifted will tend to over-investigate and this in itself will perpetuate the patient's perception of being ill.

However, I will never forget an Indian patient who had been diagnosed with renal tuberculosis and kept turning up to the clinic with very vague symptoms including mild nausea and occasional hiccoughs. There was nothing to suggest any hepatic dysfunction associated with his drug treatment; he was apyrexial and in desperation I admitted him for 'further investigation'. I spoke to his wife and her first question was 'Why has he gone so black'. She maintained that his skin colour had darkened and when we checked his biochemistry and an urgent ultrasound scan of his abdomen we found bilateral adrenal abscesses accounting for his ACTH-driven skin darkening along with his hiccough-inducing diaphragmatic irritation! There is a diagnostic tightrope that all doctors walk along with their patients and we will sometimes attribute unexplained symptoms to hysteria. Most of us will get to the other side but occasionally we will fall off along with our patients.

```
                 THE  SICK  ROOM.
           ------------------------

     If the case is serious try to find out as much as

possible from the friends beforehand in order that you may be

able to approach the patient without showing surprise and

that you need not disturb him with questions that can be

avoided.

     Knock softly at the front door.   Tread quietly.   Have

rubber heels to your boots.

     Let the greeting be kindly and hopeful, the voice low

and soothing and the hands warm.

     Try to avoid entering the room breathless.  Never

appear to be hurried or flurried.
```

THE SICK ROOM

If the case is serious try to find out as much a possible from the friends beforehand in order that you may be able to approach the patient without showing surprise and that you need not disturb him with questions that can be avoided. Knock softly at the front door. Tread quietly. Have rubber heels on your boots. Let the greeting be kindly and hopeful, the voice low and soothing and the hands warm. Try to avoid entering the room breathless. Never appear to be hurried or flurried.

There is an art in entering with a calm, earnest manner that shows interest and anxiety to learn the conditions, and in departing, with a self-satisfied demeanor that imparts confidence to the patient and the friends that you will do all that can be done as far as medical science permits.

The Medical Tactician

The majority of the public form their opinions on the care and devotion shown and the little details of routine attention. Think of everything that might be done to give the patient greater comfort. Keep clear of thinking that prescribing a drug is all you have to do.

Injunctions given under the heading of "The Interview" of course apply to the sick room. Don't forget to wash your thermometer before <u>and</u> after using it in the patient's presence.

In the sick room as at the interview in your own consulting room, the first inquiry and examination should be complete. At subsequent visits you may be able to see at a glance what the condition and progress are. But you must not dispense with asking questions about things that might be taken for granted. Such omission is likely to lead to loss of confidence and even dismissal.

Inquire in to the details of nursing. Look out for any suggestions which might add to the patient's comfort. Make considerable allowance for any rude remarks that patients may make. They are not responsible in some cases, and may apologise afterwards.

A forbearing demeanor will be appreciated by both friends and patient.

Never leave the bedside before qualifying yourself to state your opinion in clear and well-chosen language to the friends. But be very careful about what you say. It is really extraordinary how your words may be twisted.

How very true that last observation is right up to the present time. The very ill, loved-one, is seen as the helpless dependent and family and friends will feel that they are the representatives with full responsibility of ensuring that the medical staff succeed and leave 'no stone unturned' until there is full recovery. If there is any lack of clarity or conflict in information provided to the 'concerned' and the outcome from their point of view is not as expected, there will be tension between the two parties and if the patient dies and the doctor hasn't made it clear, in view of the severity of the condition, that this might be the worst case scenario, this tension is likely to erupt in to serious conflict. The latter will be due to a combination of grief, guilt as the responsible representatives of the patient, anger arising from the perception that the doctor hasn't been honest about the prognosis and someone else on the team has given conflicting information and finally a feeling of frustration that the medical profession is against them. In some cases this feeling may well be justified and a significant proportion of complaints about patient care originate from family and friends. These complaints are often the consequence of poor communication between the medical team, patient and carers.

There are, however, occasional vexatious litigants. These individuals will be hypercritical of everything that is being done and will seek conflict irrespective of the quality of care. Fortunately these situations are rare. It may be that such individuals get a 'kick' out of putting professionals under pressure – a sort of 'power trip'.

Our practitioner doesn't mention the potential for litigation but the threat must have been present. The concept of medical malpractice dates back to the 1700s when Sir William Blackstone published 'Commentaries on the Laws of England. [14] *He included the following definition of mala praxis – "Injuries caused by a physician's or an apothecary's neglect or unskillful management in violation of the trust placed in that practitioner". Several subsequent factors were identified as triggering an explosion of medical litigation. In the earlier years doctors had to compete with a wide variety of 'quacks/healers' and there were no established national standards. Our practitioner may have had to compete with such individuals and litigation was the only recourse left for patients when holding providers accountable for their actions. It wasn't long before such litigation was directed by patients and the legal profession against authentic clinicians. The main reasons for such litigation include wrong diagnosis, drugs errors or side effects, communication and surgical errors.*

In the sick room pretend not to see anything humiliating, immodest mistakes or accidental exposure.

The use of intravenous sedation for endoscopic procedures (particularly benzodiazepines) does put the patient at risk of disinhibition, during which they may become physically aggressive or may experience sexual fantasies. The latter has been a problem if the practitioner is working alone but it is well recognised that such fantasies can occur and even when there is a team in attendance during the procedure it may be difficult to persuade the patient that nothing inadvertent did occur. Fortunately, in the majority of cases, the drug has an amnesic effect as well and so any such disinhibition will not be a source of humiliation to the patient.

One of our endoscopy sisters relates an experience that their team had when the consultant was performing a colonoscopy on an 85 year old lady. Following some light Midazolam sedation and on insertion of the colonoscope, a little voice piped up, "Is that you George?" This temporarily put the operator out of action but fortunately he was able to regain his composure and the procedure was completed safely and successfully. George had long departed this world, however, my lawyers have asked me to emphasise that we have absolutely no evidence either way as to the sexual preferences of the late George.

VISITS

The frequency of visits is often a nice point to determine. If too few, the patient may complain of neglect; if too many he may suspect a desire to increase the bill. A good rule is to make as many as you conscientiously think are necessary. If numerous visits are necessary explain why. A reputation of making unnecessary visits is a bad thing to have. Do not make the visit so short as to allow the impression that you are not giving the case full attention. Do not stay longer than is necessary to give the right impression.

If a visit is made late in the day do not make the excuse that you had a long round or more important cases. Every patient thinks he is the most important. It is better to say nothing unless you can allege a confinement or accident.

It is enjoined under the heading of "The Interview" never to talk of anything till the professional side is finished. If you know the patient well, a little genial chat is often appreciated, but keep the conversation away from yourself. Lead it as far as possible to matters connected with the patient. Be a good listener. Be careful never to stay too long. It might imply that you have nothing better to do, or the patient might be bored.

Never be too busy or in too great a hurry to do your duty. If you are pressed for time do not rush into the room, throw down your hat, announce that you are very busy, make a quick examination and scribble a prescription.

The pressure of time is a serious issue in modern day medicine. A busy hospital junior doctor may receive a number of consecutive bleeps requesting action from various clinical areas and will have to prioritize on occasions. I recall one such harassed doctor being called to see the relatives of a patient who had suddenly deteriorated (not that unexpected due to his serious condition). Sister informed the doctor that the relatives were on their way and he said he would get there as soon as possible. When he arrived on the ward he saw a couple waiting outside Sister's office, ushered them in and proceeded to inform them of the sudden deterioration. Unfortunately these were not the relatives in question and had in fact arrived to take home their fully recovered father!

Economise time by being methodical and do not allow extraneous subjects to be introduced. When you have done everything needful you may remark that time is precious, if the remark is necessary.

With a garrulous patient it may be good to listen once to everything to show you are patient, and on subsequent occasions to show you have no time for other conversation.

Sometimes well-to-do people insist on unnecessary visits. Then you may gratify them, but if these are not asked for by the person who pays, let him know what is going on.

~ CHAPTER 6 ~

DIFFICULT, OBSCURE AND SERIOUS CASES

It is very unwise to diagnose where the diagnosis may turn out to be wrong. If time is likely to help, say so, and say it with emphasis, implying that the difficulty is in the nature of the case and not in your diagnostic powers. But if time is not likely to assist, it is better to suggest a consultation and have the responsibility shared. Therefore be careful about diagnosis. Make a very thorough physical examination and take the history very completely.

In early stages of the eruptive fevers the public think a diagnosis is possible. Explain emphatically that this is not possible till the local signs appear. Sometimes you can say that it is necessary to examine the urine before expressing an opinion. This appeals to most people and is generally well accepted. It gives time to think and time for fresh observation.

Errors of prognosis are often more dangerous than errors of diagnosis because the patient can easily check the error. When the time of recovery is indefinite it may work to use indefinite language, to say that it will take "some time", or that "it depends on the vitality".

A colleague of mine, when asked by the family of one of his patients what his prognosis was, made a genuinely innocent, off the cuff remark that he didn't have a crystal ball but .....
Unfortunately, they were a gypsy family and the remark wasn't best received!

Most families and some patients will want to know their prognosis. The usual question in serious cases such as cancer is 'How long have I got?' This is a potential mine field and as our practitioner rightly points out this can cause more distress than the wrong diagnosis.

This issue is addressed in an excellent overview by Christian T Sinclair. [15]

The Medical Tactician

He makes the point that an individual prognosis needs to factor in many variables such as current clinical information, diagnoses, therapeutics, social issues, functional status and of course the physician's knowledge and experience. This formulated prognosis is not necessarily the same as the true prognosis. There is evidence to suggest that patients demonstrate less anxiety and depression and are more satisfied with their doctor when the severity of the illness and life expectancy are discussed openly. His approach to the question 'How long do I have?' is to respond with, 'That is a good question, and I am glad you asked it'. This will immediately confirm that this is an important point for consideration and although it is a difficult subject it needs to be addressed. It gives time to formulate a prognosis based on the variables as above but also makes it clear to the patient that a considered response will be forth coming.

Before this prognosis is communicated it needs to be made very clear that this is an imprecise science and will be constantly changing depending on current circumstances. Once the patient and family understand the dynamic nature of the situation they will be able to accept ranges rather than a more specific figure. If the doctor, when put on the spot, states that the prognosis is about 3 months this will be repeated many times by the family and friends until it becomes a fact. Learning to be comfortable with words such as death and dying; making sure to allow for a period of silence after the prognosis is given and reinforcing that, irrespective of prognosis, there will be full continuing medical, social and spiritual care, are all crucial aspects in the management of the terminally ill.

If asked whether a case will prove fatal, say that it will depend on the possibilities of complications and that while every case presents a group of possibilities it is also surrounded by a chain of probabilities. This leaves you a margin for uncertainty.

While not holding out hopes which are false, dwell on every favourable consideration.

The Medical Tactician

In an acute case which is serious and the patient asks how serious it is, simply reply that the illness is in its early stage and that you trust he will soon be better.

In very serious cases show proper earnestness and gravity.

In hopeless cases do not give hope when there is none.

If a very ill, sane adult wishes to know his real condition, tell him he is very ill and state the grounds on which your opinion rests. But try to say it in a gentle way so as not to frighten him by taking away every hope. If there is hope, dwell on this. If there are any favourable points, mention them.

In a case where the prognosis is very bad and the patient has a tendency to ask questions that would oblige you to disclose it, be very busy examining, counting, etc., so as to give him little time for questions. Turn the conversation as quickly as possible, and so temporarily, at least, try to escape the unwelcome inquiries.

School yourself till you can prevent your thoughts, embarrassment and opinions from showing themselves in your countenance during anxieties and emergencies, so that nervous patients who are very ill cannot detect in you unfavourable reflections about themselves.

Statements to friends must be more frank than to the patient himself. While giving no false hopes, mention every favourable circumstance. The friends may know of and think of a number of things that might be done and ask why you did not do them.

Think of these things beforehand, and if the explanation is not simple, do not give it, but say decidedly that the measure would not do. Show that you are wide awake and have thought of this and that have good reasons for not using them.

RASH AND TROUBLESOME PATIENTS

Some patients may wish to do things of which you do not entirely approve. If the matter is unimportant it may be wise to humour them to some extent.

Remember that a patient's state of mind often has much to do with his recovery, and that to humour him may bring about a satisfactory condition. The case is different if the matter is serious or important. Then refuse your sanction. Should your orders still be disregarded you should consider whether it is best for you to continue on or courteously retire.

If you suspect that the cause of the disobedience is want of faith in yourself, by far the best plan is to say politely that you cannot take further responsibility.

The following is an example of a letter that might be sent.

"Dear Mrs X,

I was sorry to find today that you had gone out. This was contrary to my advice and I think it was a little injudicious. I would rather therefore not take further responsibility in the case.

With best wishes for your early recovery,

Yours very faithfully

John Smith".

CHRONIC CASES

Be frank as to time of duration. Even if you lose a case as you may, your frankness will be remembered.

Make no rash promises. If there are any encouraging circumstances, state them and really give the impression that you will do your best.

Many incurables wish you to attend them for the sake of your smile and encouragement. Do not repeat to the friends every time that you cannot cure the patient.

FEES

The amount of the fee to charge is very important but no rule can be laid down here. The rate varies so much with the class of practice and the local custom.

It is bad to charge too much; it is bad to charge too little. Patients think less of you if you do the latter. Therefore great care should be given to the subject. On the whole it is better to err on the higher scale than on the lower, but the error must not be great.

SUING

This should be avoided as far as possible. Time is taken up by it. Often the result is not satisfactory in recovering the money.

The patient frequently avenges himself by depreciating you. Generally it is better to submit to a loss. The exceptions are when the amount is large or in the case of a dissatisfied patient.

DISSATISFIED PATIENTS

If a patient has expressed dissatisfaction, send in your bill for the maximum amount. If he refuses to pay, sue without delay. In any case he will depreciate you. If you take it lying down he will boast of his moral victory and say you admitted by implication that you were wrong. A bold front minimises antagonism.

Illustrative case:

A child had enteric. Meningitis supervened and death resulted. The parents said there had been an error of diagnosis and refused to pay the bill, and boasted of their intention to the neighbours. A summons was immediately served. The money was at once paid into court.

IMPUTATIONS AGAINST PROFESSIONAL SKILL

If the imputation is slight, ignore it. If it is great protest as vigorously as possible.

DISMISSAL FROM A CASE

There are few things more humiliating than to be dismissed.

The causes are of two classes.

1. Avoidable causes

2. Unavoidable circumstances

In the first class are:-

A. Want of complete interrogation and physical examination. Want of tact.

B. The use of unpalatable drugs or expensive instruments which fail.

C. Neglect of therapeutic measures which should have been adopted.

In the second class are:-

A. Unfavourable progress of the case

B. The interference of fussy or anxious friends

If the case lies in class 1, say nothing and resolve that it shall not occur again. In A of class 2, a consultation will often preserve the case, but if in A of class 2, dismissal occurs it is better as a rule to say nothing.

In B of class 2, where you are fairly intimate with the family, it is well to say that after doing everything which you fully believed was possible, you think you have hardly been treated with courtesy.

Always send in the bill at the next quarter-day for the maximum fee. If this is not paid, promptly press for a settlement. If necessary, sue.

PATIENTS WHO ARE SLOW IN PAYING BILLS

There are cases where the account is left unpaid and in which it is undesirable to offend by pressing for a settlement.

Write at the foot of the bill, "These small amounts so often put aside and forgotten, entail extra bookkeeping and postage".

A little stronger is: - "An early settlement will be much appreciated".

Still stronger is: - "I fear this account has escaped your notice".

If an account is considerable and suing is desirable, it is better to get a solicitor to write first and add the rest later if necessary.

THE SOCIAL SIDE

Take one of the familiar puzzle pictures, a picture which represents, we will say, a house and garden and somewhere in which is concealed the outline of a human face. As you search for the face the contents of the whole picture are at a conscious focus. Suddenly you find it; and what happens? Why, as you do so, the picture disappears clean out from the focus; the face stands out with all imaginable clearness and the house and garden are no clearer than the feel of the paper between your fingers.

It is generally agreed that increased clearness of one part-contents of consciousness implies a decreased clearness of all the rest.

Associated with this law is the further psychological law that increase of clearness increases the intensity of a perception.

The above law and illustration refer to simple feelings. But what is true of these is also true of the higher compound ones with which we have to deal.

The impressions of confidence, respect, etc., on the part of the patient must be made as strong as possible. To make them strong they must be clear. To make them clear there must be an absence of other impressions, however innocent these may be.

In the article on "The Interview" it was enjoined that after professional attention, conversation should be reduced to a minimum and that the doctor would never speak about himself. In other words, that when the desired impressions have been made there should be NOTHING MORE.

In dealing with the impressions effected through the aesthetic faculties, it was shown what ought to be apparent in a doctor's house and what ought not to be apparent. That is to say, the right cords should be struck and NOTHING MORE.

These are concrete examples of the above law that clearness is proportionate to the absence of the other effects. The same law must be the guide in considering what can be gained or lost in the social side of practice.

As stated before, there is a certain ideal which patients have in mind and which you should realise as far as you are able.

The question arises, can that ideal be helped by social influences?

The opinions which it is desirable that the public should form of a practitioner are that he is:-

1.　An educated man generally

2.　A man of refinement

3.　A studious man who takes an interest in his profession.

4.　Amiable, courteous and kind.

Contrary to what is generally believed there is very little help in practice to be gained socially. There is, however, much to lose by injudicious social intercourse.

Misconceptions have arisen from seeing that men who have been successful are also socially popular. It has been assumed that the social side has been the cause of the success. In most cases it would be more correct to say, in spite of it.

There is sometimes, however, a little to be gained.

If you have a good knowledge of science and serious literature, there is no need to hide your light under a bushel.

Among intelligent people good conversational powers give the impression of professional ability which is sometimes stronger than is de facto justified.

There is therefore no harm in airing your general knowledge or good conversational powers if you have them.

On the whole the average man has much more to lose than to gain socially.

The ideal can be built up professionally, but in society it is likely to become injured.

Besides being a doctor the practitioner is also a man and the human element is apt to obtrude and distract attention from the professional one.

The two are to some extent mutually exclusive.

Avoid dinner parties at patients' houses. Do not even stop to tea if you can help it. If obliged to do so, be friendly only.

Avoid card parties where you are likely to meet patients.

Avoid expressing any political opinions. Do not take the chair at temperance meetings, etc.

In religion be straightforward. If you are not religious, do not pretend you are.

It is supposed that a country practitioner must go to church, that if he does not the clergyman will use his influence against him, etc.

The Medical Tactician

Among intelligent people good conversational powers give the impression of professional ability which is sometimes stronger than is de facto justified. There is therefore no harm in airing your general knowledge or good conversational powers if you have them.

On the whole the average man has much more to lose than to gain socially. The ideal can be built up professionally, but in society it is likely to become injured.

Besides being a doctor the practitioner is also a man and the human element is apt to obtrude and distract attention from the professional one. The two are to some extent mutually exclusive.

Avoid dinner parties at patient's houses. Do not even stop to tea if you can help it. If obliged to do so, be friendly only.

Avoid card parties where you are likely to meet patients.

Avoid expressing any political opinions. Do not take the chair at temperance meetings, etc.

In religion be straightforward. If you are not religious, do not pretend you are. It is supposed that a country practitioner must go to church, that if he does not the clergyman will use his influence against him, etc. To their credit be it said it is rarely that clergymen show themselves hostile to a non-church goer. And if they did it would be resented and a reaction would result in the practitioner's favour. Never, however, speak disrespectfully of religion. That is an entirely different matter.

Be careful never to cut people in the street or let anyone think he is beneath your notice.

Smile genially to everyone you know.

When seeing a patient at either your own house or hers there is a moment of social intercourse after the professional attention has been given.

The Medical Tactician

Then is the time to avoid spoiling the ideal which you have been trying to build up. All hobbies, amusements, and habits, must be kept in the background, however innocent these may be. A little genial pleasantry is often appreciated, but there must be nothing bordering on frivolity.

Never gossip. Never show any knowledge which might enable you to gossip.

It is a good rule never to talk of yourself. Do not boast because it is impossible to boast without being seen through, however the attempt may be.

As far as possible avoid doing business with tradesmen who are patients. If unavoidable, have no cross-accounts. Pay cash.

If asked to subscribe to charities do so with a smiling face and as liberally as your means will allow.

Do not write poetry, fiddle or sing at concerts, take part in amateur dramatic performances, or play at cricket matches. All such things would show that in the past you have spent time on non-professional matters, or that you now have the time to engage in other pursuits. The personal element is obtruded and the professional side eclipsed. The desired impressions would be made less clear as in the simple example given above.

Remember that the public and especially the female part of it have microscopic eyes, and take note of your associations and a thousand and one other facts about you. They will note your dress, actions, speech, manner, habits, and where you are found when not professionally engaged. You will be closely observed and criticised, and the verdict will be passed accordingly.

Impressions from these sources will have far more weight than any knowledge concerning your diplomas or degrees. The ideal is that you are an earnest, studious man with scientific attainments, literary tastes and correct habits.

Therefore be careful of your companions. Avoid billiard rooms, race meetings, football matches, etc.

Be courteous to all kinds of people whom you may meet. But while treating all women as sisters and all men as brothers, avoid undue familiarity with the coarse and ignorant.

Avoid a pompous and chilling manner.

A reputation for being a "nice" man is even more important than a reputation for skill. The inference is that a "nice" man is likely to do his best.

In the case of patronising social superiors, treat them with the deference due to their rank but keep them at a distance.

OBSTETRIC PATIENTS AMONG CATHOLICS

If at the birth of a child its viability is in doubt, it should be baptised at once. You or anyone else may do this, though a male catholic, if obtainable, is to be preferred.

If life is doubtful before full birth, baptise the head or presenting part. If needful, to reach the child, a syringe may be used. Use a clean glass of water.

You must use the exact words and not one word must be omitted.

Say: "I baptise thee in the name of the Father (at the word Father, pour a small quantity of the water on the child) and of the Son, (pour again) and of the Holy Ghost" (pour again). If one word is omitted, the baptism is insufficient. The water must be pure and natural and must be poured at the right words.

In catholic families you will run the risk of not being forgiven if you use forceps before the child is baptised. If this is neglected and the child is born dead, you will be blamed.

CONCLUDING REMARKS

For many years Dr Tarrasch was the greatest chess player in the world.

In 1885, then an unknown man who competed in a tournament against the keenest chess intellects of Europe, he came out second, half a point behind the first prize winner.

It was obvious from the score and from the quality of his games that a new star of the first magnitude had arisen.

In the next tournament he was repeatedly beaten by inferior players. He at once asked himself the reason. The answer was that he was suffering from delusion. Conscious of his immense powers, he had said to himself, "Because it is I, Dr Tarrasch, who is playing, the game must be won by me. I have only to make moves of some kind and I am bound to win".

His bad score aroused him from his self-deception. As he said himself, he came to the following conclusion: to win a tournament it is not sufficient to be a good player. It is also necessary to play well.

He turned this knowledge to good account and achieved the unparalleled result of competing in three successive tournaments against the finest players in the world without losing a game.

This story has a moral. To be successful in medicine it is not sufficient to have knowledge of medical tactics. It is also necessary to put this knowledge into practice. The self-deception which Dr Tarrasch discovered in himself is very likely to arise in a practitioner. A certain amount of success is apt to make a man careless. He thinks because his reputation is good it is not necessary to take the fullest pains. There is no sudden awakening such as occurs to a careless chess-player. Stationary practice against not over-strong opponents is all that may occur.

The Medical Tactician

The following considerations should be kept in mind. However skilful a medical man may be, however perfect a tactician he is, there is a centrifugal force which loses him patients.

A certain number of cases are not improved by treatment. These are more or less likely to change their doctor. The proportion averages itself and is a factor in all practices.

This centrifugal force is multiplied by any defect in tactics and reduced to a minimum by their full use.

Therefore, however successful a man may be it is necessary to exercise the fullest care in every case.

When a patient is lost, as must sometimes happen, this at least can be achieved - the next doctor need not score by comparison in care and attention.

If the centrifugal force is reduced to the lowest point and the centripetal force brought to the highest point the practice will grow till want of time sets a limit.

It is certain that personality has nothing to do with success except so far as it embraces desirable qualities. It is certain that these qualities if absent can be acquired.

It is certain that money is not necessary for success.

Sir James Paget, after making statistics of the subsequent career of a large number of students, says: - "Nothing appears more certain than that the personal character the very nature, the will of each student, had far greater force in determining his career than any help or hindrance whatever".

It is certain that however unsuccessful a man may be, a full knowledge of tactics, if out into practice, will take him upwards.

The following is an example. A newly qualified man started in practice and found himself an absolute failure. He saw that he lacked something which no text books could tell him. He became an assistant to several successful men. He carefully observed their methods. He did not learn everything but he learnt much. Then he bought a small nucleus. Today his assistant, his dispenser, and motorcar are working at full pressure.

Finally, remember that success will not be handed to you on a silver platter. It must be worked for.

The man who recognises that a small thing of no importance does not exist, has learnt a great secret of success.

~ CHAPTER 7 ~

__GENERAL SCHEME OF INTERROGATION__

Alimentary system

Appetite, thirst, fullness or pain after food, nausea, pyrosis, flatulence, state of bowels, piles, abdominal pain or tenderness.

Pyrosis is derived from the Greek for burning and refers to 'heart burn'.

Vascular System

Palpitation, dyspnoea, pain at heart.

Respiratory System

Dyspnoea, cough.

Urinary System

Quantity, frequency, pain.

Nervous System

Headache or other pains, sleep, depression of spirits, "nervousness", fears, irritability.

Generative System

Menstruation, frequency, quantity, duration, pain.

SPECIAL SCHEME OF INTERROGATION

Alimentary System

History of Present Illness.

Often difficult to get a correct answer. Ask " how long is it since you were quite well?"

Onset

Sudden or gradual. In what manner. First symptom observed.

Supposed Cause

Chill, fright, wrong diet, or excess of any kind.

Subsequent Course

Order of symptoms. Have they altered or are they the same as at first.

Loss of Weight

If any, continuous, or with intervals of increase?

Leading Symptoms

What are the particular sensations which led patient to ask advice?

On Waking

Tired or otherwise? Pain or other feelings? Nausea or vomiting? If vomiting, is it moderate and composed of mucus, bile or saliva, or is it more abundant, with acid liquid containing particles of food?

Appetite

Normal or abnormal? Complete loss or capricious? If diminished, does it return after a little food has been taken? Increased appetite? Is there a feeling of satisfaction after food? If abnormal, at all meals, or only after certain ones?

Thirst

Arrangements of Meals

Time, quantity, and kind of food? Amount of tea, coffee, alcohol, and tobacco taken? Eating or drinking between meals?

GASTRIC SENSATIONS

Feeling of Oppression or Pressure

Exact spot? Occurrence after eating or independent of food? How soon after? How long does it remain?

Fullness after Food

Present at other times as well as after food? Limited to epigastrium, or does it extend over the whole abdomen? Modified by quantity or nature of food? How soon after a meal?

Actual Pain

Character. Precise area where felt. Point of maximum intensity. Does the position change? Any connection with meals? If so, is it before, during, immediately after, or some time after? Is the pain relieved, increased or influenced by food? Does pressure increase or relieve pain? Are any spots painful to pressure? Is there any pain in the back? If so, character, position, time, relation to meals? Increased or relieved by pressure?

Flatulence

After meals, or when the stomach is empty? If after food, how long after? Any periodicity? Influenced by diet? Accompanied by other symptoms, such as headache, dyspnoea, faintness or pain in the neck?

Eructations

Slight or severe? Noiseless or explosive? Acid? Bad smell? Bitter or tasteless? Are any particles of food brought up? Occurrence during digestion or independent of it?

Vomiting and Nausea

If nausea, the time of day? If followed by vomiting? If vomiting, does it occur when the stomach is empty, or only after food? How often? Do the attacks occur in periodical groups, with intervals free from vomiting. Preceded by fullness, pain or pressure, or cramp? Does vomiting relieve the pain or discomfort? Colour, taste, smell and appearance of vomited matter? If on an empty stomach, at what time of day?

Condition of Bowels

Is there constipation? If so, do they ever act without help? If not, what is given? If motions are frequent, character, number, and influence of food?

Functional Nervous Symptoms

Tingling? Numbness, twitching, spasm, cramp? Fluxion of heat? Morbid fears? Giddiness, etc. Sleep?

Surroundings of Patient

Make a thorough inquiry as to fresh air, exercise, work, recreation, worry.

Diarrhoea

Frequency, relation to meals or special articles of food? Character of motions. Is blood or slime passed? Any straining or tenesmus?

Flatulence

History of attack. Former attacks?

VASCULAR SYSTEM

Family History

Gout, rheumatism, apoplexy, heart disease.

Personal History

Rheumatic fever, chorea, scarlatina, diphtheria?

Dyspnoea

Must the patient sit up in bed, or can he sleep lying down? When does it come on?

Praecordial Pain or Distress

Exact site and character? Does it radiate or not? If so, in what direction?

Palpitation

Relation to meals and exercise. Does the heart give a thump now and then? Sleep good or bad? Is there much dreaming? Giddiness. Is it ever present and when?

Venous distension

Do the feet swell? Cough? State of digestion. Does the nose bleed?

RESPIRATORY SYSTEM

Family History

Bronchitis, Asthma, Phthisis.

Personal History

Patient's occupation. Has he ever had enlarged glands in the neck? Is he getting thinner? Does he sweat at night?

Cough

Character, frequency. When is it worst? Accompanied by pain? Does he ever vomit with it?

Expectoration

Amount, consistence, frothy, nummular, colour, mixture of substances, blood, colourless, mixed with blood, streaked with blood, yellow, white, gummy looking, watery, thick, purulent. If blood, is it only after severe coughing? Is the blood bright and frothy, or is it dark?

Pain at Chest

Increased by breathing? Constant or not? Where situated?

Interesting lack of specific questions relating to asthma or allergies. There is the inevitable concentration on tuberculous symptoms. Nummular sputum is a thick, coherent mass of sputum in a globular shape (resembling a coin).

URINARY SYSTEM

Family History

Brights Disease, gout, apoplexy.

Personal History

Scarlatina, specific disease, lead poisoning, prolonged suppuration, gout, stone, previous renal disease. Inquire for pain in the lumbar region, acute pain shooting down into the groin, headache and vomiting, drowsiness, paralysis or fits.

Dimness of sight, dyspnoea. Does the face ever look puffy in the morning? State of bowels.

Urine

Amount. Frequency by day and night. Clear or turbid? Any blood? If so, at what period of micturition? Mixed with the urine? In clots? Are the clots moulded? If haemorrhage is paroxysmal, is there pain? Any feeling of chilliness across the loins? Weakness? Vomiting? Nausea? Joint pains? Traumatic history? Difficulty in micturition?

NERVOUS SYSTEM

Family History

Mental disease, chorea, paralysis, fits.

Patient's history

Special inquiry as to work, surroundings, past illnesses, specific disease, alcoholism.

Fits

Ask age at first fit. Any supposed cause? Describe first fit. When did they next occur? What have been the shortest and longest intervals between fits? Are they more or less frequent now? Do they occur in sleep or not? Are there any premonitions or aura? If so, what is the character? How long before loss of consciousness do they occur? Is the onset gradual or sudden? Are convulsions present? Are they general or local? Where do they begin and end? Does he fall? Has he ever hurt himself? Does he ever bite his tongue, micturate or defaecate during an attack? Are there any after symptoms, such as sleep, headache, paralysis, or mental disturbance?

General Neurasthenia

Insomnia, flushing, bad dreams, drowsiness, pain, pressure or heaviness in the head, noises in the ears, mental irritability, desire for stimulants and drugs, fear of lightning, of open or closed spaces, of being alone, of people, of contamination. Deficient mental control, lack of decision, hopelessness, sensitiveness to cold, heat, and change in the weather. Pain in the back, heaviness in the loins or limbs, local numbness or hyperaesthesiae. Difficulty in swallowing, convulsive movements in going to sleep. Feeling of profound exhaustion. Ticklishness, vague pains and flying neuralgia, local or general itching. Flashes of light, cold hands or feet. Gaping or yawning. Trembling of muscles.

BONES AND JOINTS

Family History

Tubercle, rheumatism, gout, specific disease.

Personal History

Tubercle, rheumatism, gout, specific disease, remote or recent injury. Leucorrhoea or post-partum trouble.

Pain

By day or night? If in a joint, on sudden pressure or only on movement? Starting pains at night. Influence of the weather. Does the pain shift from one joint to another?

INQUIRIES IN SOME DISEASES AND SYMPTOMS

Anaemia

Haemorrhage, menorrhagia. Past acute disease, defective hygienic surroundings. Hot rooms, want of good food regularly taken. Indigestion. Chronic gastric disease, alcoholism, plumbism, mental exhaustion, fright. Oedema of feet. When fingers are held up to light, redness of borders diminished. Headache, spinal and intercostal neuralgia. Muscular weakness, mental weakness and irritability.

Rickets

Conditions of feeding, ability to walk or stand. Age at which walking began. Previous health. Sweating, especially about the head. Are clothes thrown off at night? Is the head rubbed on the pillow? Was dentition late? General tiredness, crying on being moved. Diarrhoea. Cough, convulsions, laryngismus. Premature birth.

Rheumatism

History of Rheumatism. Chorea in family? Previous attacks? Delirium? Sleep? Exposure to cold and wet?

Rheumatoid Arthritis

Debilitating causes. Haemorrhage. Mental depression. Starvation. Dampness. Heredity.

Headache

Situation. General or local? Character. Dull, heavy, throbbing, shooting, sense of fullness, constant, intermittent, recurrent, periodical. Intensity. Variability. Sense of movement and change of position, of light and sound. Mode of onset. Previous attacks. Soreness or tenderness at spots. Vomiting? History of neurosis in patient or family? Of phthisis or struma? Inquire for overwork, sleeplessness, want of food, error of diet, constipation. Are disorders of sight present? Does patient see sparks, colours, stars, zig-zags?

Vertigo

Time of occurrence? At waking? Alcoholism, excessive smoking. Anaemia. Dyspepsia, exposure to sun.

Are objects stationary? Do objects appear to move, up and down, horizontally, approaching or receding? Increased or relieved by movement or position?

Neuralgia

Onset. Sudden or gradual? Preceded by general or local disturbances? Severity, frequency and character of pain. Effect of heat and cold. History of hysteria, epiplepsy, traumatism, specific disease, gout, rheumatism. Anaemia, cold, mental anxiety. Herpes Zoster.

Trigeminal – Tender points: 1) Supra-orbital. 2) Palpebral, at junction of nasal bone and cartilage. 3) Ocular, at inner angle of orbit.

Sciatic – Tender points, course of nerve and branches, gluteal region, back of thigh. Calcaneal and malleolar branches. Also behind trochanter.

Intercostal neuralgia – Constant or shooting. Painful points. 1) Vertebral. 2) Outer margin of trapezius. 3) Sternal.

Chorea

Previous attacks? If so, one sided, and which side? Manner of beginning? Nervous system generally. History of school life. Headaches. Rheumatism. Mental symptoms.

Hysteria

Loss of energy, attacks, fits or convulsions. If any, under what circumstances? Headaches, neuralgia, infra-mammary, or of nerve V. Local anaesthesia, functional paralysis, spasm.

Herpes Zoster

History. Date of onset of symptoms. Tender points. Did pain precede eruption? Recent use of arsenic?

Arsenic when considered in its very toxic form referred to Arsenic Trioxide or 'White Arsenic' which was available in large quantities as a by-product of the smelting process of various metals. The major rat problem offered one way of disposing of this by-product and when the public became aware of its serious toxic effects, the additional use in the disposing of unwanted humans soon caught on! This was further stimulated by the upsurge in the life insurance business! It was the ideal poison because it was colourless and tasteless. I presume our practitioner had to be aware of any signs that might indicate accidental or non-accidental poisoning. Arsenic could produce nodular skin lesions which I presume had some characteristics in common with the skin eruptions seen in Herpes Zoster.

Interrogation concerning children

How many other children? Any dead and of what? Where does the patient come in the family? Any miscarriages? If so, when? Health of father's and mother's family? Mother's health during pregnancy? A full-time child? Was the labour normal? Was the child breast-fed? If not, how was it fed? What food does it get now? Had it any rash or snuffles? Time of teething? Of walking? What is the usual state of digestion and bowels? Previous illnesses? Fits? Dates. Diarrhoea, vomiting, sore throat, measles, scarlatina, whooping cough?

~ CHAPTER 8 ~

PHYSICAL EXAMINATION

The order of examining the various systems is immaterial, but some order should be chosen and kept to, with an exception. The system which is most affected should be taken first.

The Abdomen

Abdominal examinations should not be made in women, unless the symptoms require it, or unless the patient is nervous about a 'tumour', or if, with abdominal signs, the progress of the case is not good. If there is no urgency, and reluctance is shown, postpone it. With men it should be more a matter of routine in any case of consequence, as severe dyspepsia.

One can imagine our practitioner avoiding any examination of his female patient's abdomen as she appears rather over weight and he doesn't want to offend her sensitivities. He then notes that the 'progress of the case is not good' and finally examines her to find a large abdominal mass is the cause of her protuberant abdomen!

Inspection

Is there bulging? If so, note whether general, and position, if local. Does the swelling move with or independently of respiration?

Pulsation in the gastric region may be caused by 1) Distension of the right ventricle, 2) Venous pulsation of the liver, 3) Aortic pulsation, (common in nervous people, especially women), 4) Tumour or aortic aneurysm.

Palpation

Patient should be on his back, knees drawn up, and shoulders a little raised.

Tell him to keep his mouth open, and to breathe quietly. Divert him by talking. Ordinarily use one hand only, which should be warm. Let the hand rest a moment on the skin before beginning. Palpate each region systematically. Avoid poking with the finger tips. Use gentle movement from the metacarpo-pharyngeal joints. During expiration follow the wall and gently rotate with the fingers.

In obscure cases examine the patient in a hot bath. The patient gets in at 100F. Raise rapidly to 110F. Complete relaxation usually now occurs, but sometimes it is necessary to go to 120F.

Percussion

Percuss in the usual manner, and also by flicking, to detect slight dullness. To flick, press forefinger of left hand firmly on abdomen, palmar surface upwards. Flick with middle finger of right, released from thumb.

Transmitted thrill from fluid in peritoneum

Patient on back. Press one hand over lumbar region. Tap opposite lumbar region sharply with other hand. In fat people, to avoid getting a thrill through abdominal walls, get an assistant to put his hand with the edge firmly on the wall in the middle line.

The size of the kidney cannot be made out by percussion. In all cases of abdominal enlargement, measure circumference at umbilicus for future comparison.

In rectal examination, remember that haemorrhoids are not palpable

THE VASCULAR SYSTEM – Inspection

Form of paecordia (Bulging, flatness)

Form of surrounding parts (Bulging)

Praecordial movements – Apex beat, force, position, extent. Diffuse pulsation. Pulsation at base of heart.

Movements outside praecordial region

At episternal notch. (Aneurysm. Large Throidea Ima, abnormal origin of right subclavian. Differentiate by palpation)

The thyroidea ima artery ascends in front of the trachea to the lower part of the thyroid gland, which it supplies. It varies greatly in size and when present, arises from the brachiocephalic trunk (innominate artery).

Movements outside sterno-mastoid

Carotid pulsation. Venous pulse in jugular, (from back pressure on right side of heart).

Pulsation in thorax outside praecordia

Aneurysm, pulsating empyema, malignant tumour.

In Epigastrium

Pulsation, (systolic or delayed). Systolic depression, (from adhesions or old pericarditis).

To Determine Whether Pulsation Is Expansile

Place flags on each side of tumour. If expansile, the free ends will recede. Improvised flags. Fix piece of stiff ointment to straw or bristle, 3 inches long. Stick ointment on skin. Or pass a pin through a piece of strapping, with head on sticky side. Stick strapping to skin. Veins of thoracic walls. Note if dilated. (Impeded right side. Portal obstruction).

Palpation

How to palpate – Have a patient lying on his back. Stand at patient's head on right side. Place hand (warm) with palm over base and fingers directed to apex. Don't dig finger tips into intercostals spaces.

135

When pulsation is detected, determine exact locality with pulp of fingers. Apex beat may be impalpable from weak heart, emphysema, thick chest walls. Use palpation to confirm inspection, to detect thrills. Note whether these are presystolic, systolic or diastolic.

Palpation at Episternal Notch

Try to avoid hurting the patient. If pulsation is present, try to press fingers below it to diagnose aneurysm from abnormal right subclavian.

Palpation in Epigastrium

Press gently, but firmly, over left costal margin to diagnose pulsation of right ventricle from pulsating liver.

Percussion

1. Keep pleximeter, or finger, in firm contact with chest walls.
2. Keep axis of pleximeter parallel to edge of organ, and line of percussion at right angles to this.
3. In defining a boundary, percuss from the resonant to the less resonant.
4. Don't give more than two or three blows at a time. Otherwise discomfort is caused.
5. Deliver stroke from wrist and finger joints, not from the elbow. Terminal phalanx should be at right angles to metacarpals. Strike perpendicularly. When the stroke has been given, raise striking finger at once from pleximeter.

Auscultation

Don't use a stethoscope with a metal chest-piece. It strikes cold. If using a single one, beware of pressing more than gently. Listen with a double one also.

Listen for haemic murmurs in second left intercostal space, just external to the pulmonary area.

To hear the bruit de diable in chlorosis, press very gently over the clavicular head of the sterno-mastoid.

R L Thomas writes about Chlorosis in the 'Eclectic Practice of Medicine', 1907. He considers it to be a form of primary anaemia predominantly affecting females from around 14 – 20 years of age. It was more common in bad housing or work conditions with little sunshine and in those that ate 'hastily, improperly prepared food'. There seemed to be an association with TB but this might just be a function of lower socio-economic life style. The patients would take on a greenish-yellow hue and the symptoms reported would all be in keeping with severe anaemia. There would also be associated gastric symptoms with anorexia and acid reflux. Cardiac auscultation would reveal a soft systolic murmur, heard most pronounced over the pulmonary area and a continuous murmur or venous hum over the veins of the neck, otherwise known as 'bruit de diable' or 'Nun's murmur' but I haven't been able to discover why. The sclera were said to take on a bluish appearance. This tends to occur in hyperdynamic states such as anaemia or thyrotoxicosis and results from increased blood flow through the internal jugular veins especially on the right side. It will disappear with jugular vein compression.

I S Loudon [16] produced a comprehensive overview of the mysterious condition of Chlorosis and divided the history of the condition into 4 phases:

1) *Before 1750 it was described as the 'disease of virgins' a disorder due to 'unrequited love'.*
2) *Between around 1750-1850 it was believed to be related to amenorrhoea.*
3) *After 1850 it was considered to be a special form of anaemia which was peculiar to young women.*
4) *From 1900-20 the diagnosis seems to have disappeared.*

He speculates that a number of the clinical features of Chlorosis would be in keeping with anorexia nervosa.

The Pulse

Examine with forearm pronated. Make a habit of feeling both radials. Aortic aneurysm or abnormal position of vessel might be detected.

To determine calibre

Empty by firm pressure, and try to measure breadth in flattened state. If this is impossible, let blood return below finger, and note size of artery. Caution: be sure you are feeling the radial. It may wind round to the back unusually high, and the superficialis volae may run in the site of the radial.

To ascertain state of walls

Flatten vessel and slip skin up and down over it. In health, the wall can rarely be felt. In disease, thickening, calcification, tortuosities or dilatations may be discovered.

To measure maximum pressure or force

Use three fingers; press firmly with the one nearest wrist, to prevent recurrent pulsation from palmar arch. Adjust pressure of middle finger till pulse is most distinct. Then note the amount of pressure required by the finger above to stop pulse felt by middle finger.

To test for maximum pressure

Roll the artery from side to side between the beats. If pressure is low, the vessel may not be felt. If high, it may feel like a whipcord.

The Medical Tactician

RESPIRATORY SYSTEM

Inspection of chest – deviation from normal

Symmetrical chest showing a proclivity to disease (Phthinoid) – *an obsolete term for wasting or consumptive. A long narrow chest, the lower ribs being more oblique than usual and sometimes reaching almost to the crest of the ilium, with the scapulae projecting backward, the manubrium sterni depressed, and with the sternal angle sharper than normal; such a chest was once considered indicative of pulmonary tuberculosis.*

The alar chest:

Long and shallow thorax, long neck, prominent throat. Vertebral borders of scapulae project, shoulders droop.

Flat chest:

Costal cartilages more or less straight.

Symmetry with indicated past disease

Rachitic chest:

Vertical groove at junction of bone and cartilage

Pigeon breast:

Obstruction to inspiration in young life.

Harrison's sulcus:

Commences at level of xiphisternum. Passes outwards and a little downwards (same cause as Pigeon breast).

The Medical Tactician

<u>Symmetry with indication of disease</u>

Emphysema:

Ribs less oblique. Spine too concave forwards. Sternum too arched. Barrel shape. Note that kyphosis simulates emphysematous forms.

Bilateral hollow:

Phthisis

<u>Unilateral changes</u>

Enlargement:

Fluid or gas in pleura. Tumour in lung.

Diminution:

Phthisis, adhesions, collapse from bronchial obstruction.

<u>Local changes</u>

Bulging:

Emphysema, effusion, tumour, heart disease.

Shrinking:

Phthisis, adhesions

Funnel shaped depression in lower part of midline:

Congenital, respiratory obstruction in infancy, shoemakers

(*It was felt that the chest may become misshapen as a consequence of posture in certain employments and trades:*

thus shoemakers have a depression at the lower end of the sternum).

Respiratory Movements

Rate

Ratio to pulse

Rhythm

Type – thoracic, abdominal

Local deficiency in expiration (Phthisis, lobar pneumonia)

Inspiratory indrawing

Expiratory bulging

Measurement and Palpation

Use cyrtometer to measure circumference at nipples, in full inspiration and full expiration.

Nature of Respiratory Movements

Fix finger tips at patient's sides. Make radial borders of thumbs, meet in middle line. Keep hands rigid. Direct full inspiration. Distance of departure of thumbs shows extent of expansion of each side.

Tactile Vocal Fremitus

Percussion

Ordinary percussion.

With tuning fork. To make out limits of lungs. Place plate end of vibrating fork on interspace in front of chest. Listen with stethoscope posteriorly.

Auscultation

Direct patient to breathe through nose, regularly, and very deeply, but not noisily. To suppress adventitious sounds on a hairy chest, moisten the skin.

Cautions: Crepitations at the base may mean nothing. If a patient has been breathing quietly for some hours, and especially if he has been lying down, a few crepitations at the apex may mean nothing.

Cog-wheel respiration is not to be relied on as diagnostic.

Bronchophony and pectoriloquy. Caution: See that the patient's lips are not directed to the stethoscope.

NERVOUS SYSTEM

Memory

Distinguish between memory of recent, and that of former events. Ask the patient what time he got up, and what he had for breakfast, etc.

In neurasthenia, recollections of old occurrences may be good, and that of recent ones, bad. If the memory is deficient, attach less importance to the history.

Speech

Lalling (*a form of stammering when the speech is almost unintelligible*). Baby speech. Get the patient to read aloud. In lalling, the difficult consonants are dropped.

The Medical Tactician

<u>Staccato Speech</u>

The patient speaks slowly, and syllable by syllable.

<u>Slurring</u>

As in intoxication. Typically seen in G.P.

I presume this refers to General Paralysis of the Insane. This was a neuro- psychiatric disorder affecting the brain and central nervous system, caused by syphilis infection. The patient usually presented with psychotic symptoms of sudden onset. It is now rare in most developed countries. It was first described as a distinct disease in 1822 and predominantly affected people in second to fourth decades. By 1877, for example, the superintendent of an asylum for men in New York reported that in his institution this disorder accounted for more than 12% of the admissions and more than two percent of the deaths. Our practitioner is therefore likely to have come across this condition.

<u>Syllable Stumbling</u>

Ask the patient to say 'utterly erroneous error'. Some syllables are repeated, and some letters misplaced.

<u>Aphasia</u>

Comprises loss of power to talk; inability to write; word deafness; word blindness. Combinations of these are common.

<u>Test with Spoken Speech</u>

Ascertain if the hearing is good. Ask patient to shut his eyes, etc. If hearing is present test knowledge of nouns by asking him to touch something, then his knowledge of verbs by asking him to do something. If these tests are passed, there is no word deafness.

The Medical Tactician

Observations to be Made

If the vocabulary is very limited, note the words. If the word, or phrase, is repeated, note it. If the vocabulary is considerable, note lalling, slurring, etc, that is, the power of articulation. Test him with pronouns, long words as 'deliberate animosity'. Show him common objects, and ask him to name them. If he is dumb, ask him to show on his fingers the number of syllables in each word. If he cannot do this, he has forgetfulness of words. Sometimes he omits some syllables, or substitutes others. If he calls a table a chair, etc., he has Paraphasia. Note whether he is aware of this, or whether he tries to correct a mistake. Ask him to repeat words after you. If he can do this, try to find out if he understands what he is saying.

Written Speech

Test the sight. If this is good, write simple questions or commands on paper, and show to him. If no response, there is word blindness. Ask him to write his name. If he can do this, ask him to write down the answer to the question, "how much do 2 and 3 make?" If he has word deafness, ask him in writing. If the right hand is paralysed, ask him to write with the other. If he writes well, ask him to write an account of his illness, and note whether he uses a wrong word at times (Paragraphia), or whether there is repeated use of a particular word. Can he write to dictation or copy? If so, does he understand the meaning? Does he shake his head for "no", or nod it for "yes"? Does he shake his head for "yes".

Write down	2	2
	2	2
	4	5

Ask him which is right.

Can he recognise common objects? Put a pencil and other things beside him, then ask him to write something down. If he selects the wrong article or cannot recognise friends, he is mind blind.

CRANIAL NERVES

The First

Test smell with bottles of oil of cloves, of oil of peppermint, and of tincture of assafoetida. Test each nostril separately, and ask what it is. Don't use Ammonia, this is recognised partly by the fifth. If loss of smell has existed two years, it will not return.

The Second

Field of vision: For ordinary purposes this can be tested:-

Sit opposite the patient, about 18 inches from him. To test his right eye, ask him to cover his left eye and look at your left eye. Stare at his right eye, your own right eye being covered. Move your fore-finger in a plane midway between his face and yours. Hold the finger first at a remote part of the plane, where you cannot see it. Gradually approach the centre. Ask the patient to let you know when he can see the finger. Note position at which he can see it, and at which you can see it. Test upwards and downwards, to right and to left. Test the other eye similarly.

The Third

Paralysis of the third; ptosis, is often partial. To estimate the amount, eliminate the action the occipito-frontalis by pushing this down to keep the eyebrows level. Then ask the patient to look up. Extent of raising of lid shows strength of levator.

The Medical Tactician

Examination of the Pupils

The size frequently varies in health. If dilated, often a sign of nervous exhaustion. But remember that in myopia dilatation is normal. Slight inequality of pupils may mean nothing. If one is larger than the other, the less mobile one should be considered the abnormal. Note the shape. Irregularities are often an early symptom of G.P. (*Argyll-Robertson pupils of Syphilis*).

The Fifth

Testing motor functions:

Keep your hands on temporals and masseters, and ask the patient to clench his teeth. The muscles should stand out equally on each side. On opening the mouth, the jaw deviates to the paralysed side, pushed by the healthy pterygoid.

Testing sensory functions:

Lesions affect the taste. Test by placing sugar and quinine on the tongue. Ask what they are.

The Seventh

Ask the patient to shut his eyes as tightly as possible. Note the total or partial failure on the affected side. Try to open forcibly closed eyes against a patient's resistance. Ask him to whistle, smile, or show his teeth. Ask if there is a hypersensitiveness to sounds. If this is present, the lesion is before entering the aqueduct, causing paralysis of the stapedius.

The Ninth

Rarely paralysed alone. Test the taste in the posterior part of the tongue. Tickle the back of the pharynx, and note if any reflex is present.

The Tenth

If both palatine branches are affected, there is regurgitation through the nose on swallowing. Pronunciation is affected. These symptoms are not observed in unilateral paralysis. Depress the tongue with a depressor. Ask the patient to say "ah". Note whether both sides of the palate arch upwards. Note the uvula. If one side is paralysed, that will remain flat and immobile. The median raphe will be pushed to the other side. In bilateral paralysis the whole palate remains motionless. Bilateral paralysis of superior laryngeal branch causes hoarse deep voice, and makes high notes impossible.

The Eleventh

Ask the patient to shrug his shoulders against resistance. If the sterno-mastoid is affected, there is difficulty in rotation of chin to opposite side.

The Twelfth

Ask the patient to put out his tongue, move it from side to side, to lick his cheeks. Note deviation, wasting, tremor or twitching.

MOTOR FUNCTIONS

Flexors of fingers

Note power to squeeze your hand.

Opponens Pollicis

Ask the patient to touch the tip of his little finger with the point of his thumb.

Adductor of Thumb

Ask him to grasp a book between fore-finger and thumb, keeping both in the same plane.

Flexors of Wrist

Hand being held palm upwards, ask him to bring the points of his fingers towards the front of his forearm.

Extensors of Wrist

Patient's palm being downwards, grasp his wrist, and ask him to bend the hand up backwards as far as possible.

Supinator Longus

With arm midway between pronation and supination, ask him to flex forearm against resistance. If muscle is healthy it will stand out prominently at upper part.

Biceps

Elbow being at side, ask for flexion while opposing at wrist. A healthy biceps will stand out prominently.

Triceps

Test similarly

Deltoid

If paralysed, inability to lift arm straight out at right angles.

Pectorals

Ask patient to stretch his arms out in front of him. Then ask him to clap his hands against resistance. Note contraction of both muscles.

Serratus Magnus

Ask patient to push against resistance. If muscle is paralysed, the scapula will project when he pushes.

Muscles of Trunk

If a patient, lying on his back, is unable to rise without using his arms, there is weakness of the abdominal muscles. To test muscles of back, lay patient on his face, and ask him to raise his head by extending neck and back. If the back muscles are healthy, they will stand out.

Extensors of Knee

Bend up knee, press with your hand on the sole of foot. Ask patient to straighten it out.

Flexors of Knee

Lay him on his face. Ask him to flex against resistance.

Extensors of Thigh

Lift his foot off the bed, and ask him to extend against resistance.

Flexors of Thigh

With extended knee ask him to raise the limb.

Adductors and Abductors of Thigh

Test against resistance.

Rotators of Thigh

Place patient on his face. Bend knee to a right angle. Ask him to roll the limb in or out against resistance.

TESTING MUSCULAR COORDINATION

Upper Limb

Ask the patient with bandaged eyes to touch the point of his nose, first with one then with the other forefinger.

Lower Limb

Ask him to walk along a straight line, (a crack in the floor, or the edge of the carpet). If he cannot walk, ask him to touch the dorsum of one foot, with the great toe of the other.

REFLEXES

When knee jerks cannot be obtained without "re-inforcement". To "reinforce", ask the patient to hook the fingers of the two hands together, and to pull as hard as ever he can. Knee jerks may be obtained.

THE LOCOMOTOR SYSTEM

Long Bones

Shaft. Press hand along noting tenderness or thickening. Thickening most likely to be found on anterior surface of tibia and lower ends of radius and ulna. Indicates periostitis, possibly specific.

(Syphilis remains high on the differential diagnostic list at the beginning of the 20th century).

End of Bones

Look for general enlargement a sign of rickets, or nodulation of margin as in rheumatoid arthritis.

JOINTS

Inspection

Position, form, redness.

Palpation

Heat, tenderness, fluctuation

On Moving

Note mobility, pain, grating. Look for thickening, bogginess of synovial membrane. When possible, feel articular surface for thickening or lipping.

VERTEBRAL COLUMN

Look for projection of spines. If any, count to the vertebra prominens, or twelfth dorsal, (if the last rib can be distinctively felt). Note general curvature, lateral or antero-posterior. Ask patient to stoop down. Note mobility, and exact site of pain, if present. Search for tender points with the hand. These can be more readily found by drawing a hot sponge down the column. Look for deep-seated tenderness by "punching" the spine gently with the fist from above, downwards. Mark point and verify by repeating process from below upwards. In suspected early caries, press patient's head down when he is erect.

I suspect that caries, when used in this context, refers to a progressive destruction of any bone structure, including the skull, ribs and other bones, or the teeth. This might be due to osteomyelitis and perhaps our practitioner was thinking about mastoiditis or osteomyelitis of the upper spine.

THE SKULL

If swelling is detected, note whether a hard rim can be found, and if this disappears on steady pressure. Can the swelling be moved? Is there a hole on the skull, or not (to diagnose extravasation from depressed fracture).

In children, examine fontanelles and sutures. Search for unossified area, (craniotabes).

Tabes means wasting of the body or part of it. This term was often found on death certificates of young children and probably indicated TB. Craniotabes can be a normal finding in infants and may occur in up to one third of newborns, especially premature infants. It is a harmless finding unless associated with other problems, e.g. rickets and osteo- genesis imperfecta. It is demonstrated by pressing the bone along suture lines where it may pop in and out, similar to pressing on a Ping-Pong ball.

Note any tender spots, tapping gently all over the surface. These may be found in neuralgia, intra-cranial tumour, and in inflammatory conditions of the bones and membranes.

GAITS

The spastic."Sticky gait". (Lateral sclerosis. Hemiplegic gait).

The ataxic. Stamping.

Reeling. (cerebellar disease).

Festination. (Paralysis agitans).

Literally shaking palsy and refers to Parkinson's Disease.

Waddling.

(Congenital dislocation. Pseudo-hypertrophic paralysis)

THE SKIN AND HAIR

Certain discolourations may be suspected of being tuberculous. Press them with any piece of glass e.g. a lens. If the colour disappears, it is not tubercle.

Pediculi. Nits slide along the hair. Epithelium comes off. Nits are placed first near the scalp. Therefore the higher up on the hair, the longer they have been there.

CHILDREN PHYSICAL EXAMINATION

This often presents difficulties. Help from the patient is usually absent, and strong opposition may be present.

During interrogation of the mother, try to gain the child's confidence. Talk to him. Learn his name or pet name. If very young, give him the stethoscope to play with, in order that he may not be afraid of it later. If old enough to eat sweets, give him one. It is a very wise plan to keep a stock, and well worth the trouble. A little thing like this may seem unimportant. But popularity with the child will be appreciated by the mother, and will be talked about.

Extreme gentleness and unlimited patience are necessary. Before the child is undressed, note the face, the colour of the lips, and whether the alae nasi are acting.

I think our practitioner means checking whether the Levator Alae Nasi are acting. These are considered to be accessory muscles of respiration in that they flare the nostrils to increase air entry and may indicate a degree of respiratory failure. Particularly noticeable in horses after a race!

At this stage also count the respirations by watching the movements of the abdomen.

To count the pulse, let the mother hold the child's hand. Then slip your own over the mother's. If the child has begun to cry, it is useless to count, for the rate may be 20 above normal. The character of the pulse is of little value in children.

System cannot be well followed. Rely more on inspection and palpation than on auscultation and percussion.

153

Strip the child, and place him in a blanket on the mother's knee. The anterior fontanelle should be closed between the fifteenth month and the second year. If open after the second year suspect rickets. Too early closing may mean idiocy.

At the beginning of the 20th century a classification system for mental retardation was proposed. Individuals with a mental age of less than 3 years were identified as idiots; imbeciles had a mental age of 3 to 7 years, and morons had a mental age of 7 to 10 years. The term "idiot" was used to refer to people having an IQ below 30.

The fontanelle should pulsate distinctively, and be neither sunken nor elevated. It is normally tense when the child is crying.

Look for bosses on the frontal and parietal bones (Rickets). These also occur in specific disease, craniotabes in children, and as rheumatic nodules in older.

Shape of Skull

Box-shaped in rickets, globular in hydrocephalus.

Long Bones

Examine for thickening along the shafts; also for tenderness. (Scurvy, specific disease or suppurative periostitis). Enlarged epiphyses (rickets) best seen at the junction of ribs and sternum, or at the wrist.

The term 'Rachitic Rosary', particularly in children, referred to the row of beadlike prominences at the junction of ribs and its cartilages in rickets.

Rheumatic nodules vary in size, from a pin head to a pea. Found in deep fascia where it covers superficial bones, and in sheaths of tendons. Look specially over olecranon and patella. If present they are pathognomonic of rheumatism.

Examine the vertebral column.

Take the temperature in the groin, in older children in the mouth.

Thorax and Abdomen

Inspect chest, next palpate, (with warm hand). Auscultation and percussion last. Percuss very lightly.

Leave examination of mouth and throat to the last. Begin with looking at the tongue. In little babies gentle pressure over the chin may open the mouth. Or a drop of milk on the lip may cause the child to lick it off and show the tongue. It may be necessary to press the lower lip on the teeth. Sometimes the nostrils have to be compressed.

Once the mouth is open, inspect the mucous membrane for thrush.

In suspected measles look for Koplik's spots. These are red with a bluish white speck in the centre of each. Observe in strong sunlight, not in bright artificial light. They may precede the eruption by three to five days.

If it's necessary to pass the finger in the naso-pharynx to examine for adenoids, biting the finger can be prevented as follows:-

Stand on right side of child. Pass left arm around head. Press cheek in between upper and lower teeth. Remember that examination is painful, and that you will make an enemy of the child. If enlarged tonsils and adenoid symptoms are present, do not examine.

In auscultating, remember that children's chests convey sounds well, that abnormal sounds caused on one side may be heard on both.

To test knee jerks, note that the tendon lies on the outer side, and may be easily missed.

To test light perception in babies, observe if the eyes follow a candle held near, or threaten the cornea by bringing the finger near and note if the child winces.

In examining the ear, don't use a speculum in young children. (See section on diseases of the ear).

GENERAL REMARKS ON ROUTINE

Some of the above is difficult to memorise. The interrogation on the alimentary system is formidable. Until it is mastered, the following plan may be adopted. Have the headings typed on the left hand side of pages of foolscap.

The patient will think this is done to save time. The cheapest way to get duplicated typed matter is to apply to one of the typewriter companies, or to the Roneo Duplicator Co. Holborn, London.

There are many important rules to follow in tactics. One of the most essential is to make the most complete examination and interrogation. It inspires confidence; it gives the impression of personal and professional interest. It is a strong and legitimate means of gaining reputation. Its absence is one of the avoidable causes of dismissal from a case.

If patients are worth having, it is worth while taking trouble to get them. It is a certainty that the time consumed will repay itself well.

~ EPILOGUE ~

This snapshot in to the past provides us with an overall flavour of the day to day strivings of a medical practitioner to be successful in his practice some 100 years ago. The emphasis is very biased to making a good impression in order to make a good living. However, there are many areas in which we see his compassion for patients rather than just considering them as a means to a financial end.

When comparing modern day medical practice with his views we see a number of fascinating differences. He emphasises the importance of influencing women as it is their word of mouth that will enhance his reputation. At the same time, however, he sees them as being "much more impressionable through the emotional and aesthetic faculties." One gets the impression that he is much more on his guard when dealing with women and he takes pains to avoid asking them indelicate questions when taking a history and may skip certain parts of the physical examination to avoid any embarrassment. "Abdominal examinations should not be made in women, unless the symptoms require it."

The paternalistic approach with patients is very much in evidence. There seems to be a tendency to avoid, where possible, the breaking of any bad news and a reluctance to discuss the mechanisms by which the limited available therapies work.

We get an insight in to the class system pertaining at that time. "With working people a greater heartiness in the tone of voice is desirable, while avoiding any undignified familiarity. Such patients are often embarrassed at meeting their 'betters', afraid that they are giving trouble or intruding." There is an early indication of therapeutic restriction when he notes that Digalen might be appropriate in some patients who can afford it.

The high awareness of tuberculosis and syphilis reminds us of the prevalence of such diseases during those years and it is a sobering thought when we consider the persisting scourge of tuberculosis even though a century has passed.

Asthma is only briefly referred to although the condition had been recognised for centuries. Asthma was considered to be a nervous disorder throughout most of its history. Conditions such as scarlatina, whooping cough, measles, chorea, scurvy, rickets, lead and arsenic poisoning, were much more prevalent then.

More is written about neurasthenia and I suspect a lot of our practitioner's experience revolved around the differential between neurosis and disease. There would have been much greater pressure in light of childhood mortality rates and a lot of his expertise would have involved dealing with bereaved parents.

I think his need to impress patients with his attention to detail, 'cleverness' and professionalism, teaches us a lot about the general practice of medicine at that time and there are many useful observations that ring true in today's doctor-patient relationships, even allowing for a gap of 100 years.

~ REFERENCES ~

1   Professor Anne Digby

     The Evolution of British General Practice 1850 -
     1948. Published by Oxford University Press 1999

2   Prof D G Kemperer.

     Elements of the Clinical Diagnosis. 1899 London:
     MacMillan

3   Clemens von Pirquet

     Klinische Studien über Vakzination und vakzinale
     Allergie. Münchener medizinische Wochenschrift,
     1906, 53, 1457-1458.

4   Samuel Meltzer

     Journal of the American Medical Association,
     Chicago, 1910, 55: 1021-1024.

     The work of John Auer and Paul Adin Lewis (1879
     -1929) led Meltzer to the conclusion that bronchial
     asthma was due to anaphylaxis, although he did not
     appreciate that all cases of asthma were so caused.

5   Bernardino Ramazzini

     His book on occupational diseases, *De Morbis
     Artificum Diatriba,* (*Diseases of Workers*), 1713.

6   J Munroe Campbell

     Acute symptoms following work with hay. BMJ
     1932,2,1143

7   Patient Choice

        http://www.nhs.uk/choiceintheNHS/Yourchoices/all
        aboutchoice/Pages/Allaboutchoice.aspx

8   Silas Weir Mitchell

        Doctor and Patient. Philadelphia and London:

        J.B.Lippincott Co., 1888.

9   Charlotte Perkins

        The Yellow Wallpaper. *The New England
        Magazine*, Volume 11, Issue 5, January 1892.

10   Anton J M de Craen et al.

        Placebos and placebo effects in medicine: historical
        overview. Journal of the Royal Society of Medicine.
        Vol 92, October 1999

11   Haygarth J
.
        Of the Imagination, as a Cause and as a Cure of
        Disorders of the Body;
        Exemplified by Fictitious Tractors, and Epidemical
        Convulsions. Bath: Crutwell, 1801

12   R Adler and N Cohen.

        Behaviourally conditioned immuno-
        suppression. Psychosomatic Medicine, Vol 37,
        Issue 4, 333-340.

13   Pert CB, Ruff MR, Weber RJ, Herkenham M.

Neuropeptides and their receptors: a psychosomatic network. J Immunol. 1985 Aug;135(2 Suppl):820s - 826s.

14   Commentaries on the Laws of England are an influential 18th-century treatise on the common law of England by Sir William Blackstone.

Published by the Clarendon Press at Oxford, 1765-1769. The work is divided into four volumes, on the rights of persons, the rights of things, of private wrongs and of public wrongs.

15   Christian T Sinclair

Communicating a Prognosis in Advanced Cancer. The Journal of Supportive Oncology - Vol 4, Number 4, April 2006.

16   I S L Loudon

Chlorosis, anaemia, and anorexia nervosa. British Medical Journal. Vol 281, 20-27, Dec 1980.